Hypertension Management for the Primary Care Clinician

Hypertension Management

for the Primary Care Clinician

Alan H. Mutnick, Pharm.D., R.Ph., FASHP
Assistant Director for Clinical Services
University of Virginia Health System
Charlottesville, VA

Tina M. Hisel, Pharm.D., BCPS
Assistant Professor (Clinical)
University of Iowa College of Pharmacy
Iowa City, IA
Broadlawns Family Practice Residency Program
Des Moines, IA

Jacqueline D. Joss, Pharm.D.
Clinical Pharmacy Specialist, Ambulatory Care
Good Samaritan Regional Medical Center
Samaritan Health Services
Corvallis, OR

Beth Bryles Phillips, Pharm.D., BCPS
Clinical Pharmacy Specialist, Ambulary Care
University of Iowa Hospitals and Clinics
Iowa City, IA

American Society of Health-System Pharmacists®
Bethesda, Maryland

Any correspondence regarding this publication should be sent to the publisher, American Society of Health-System Pharmacists, 7272 Wisconsin Avenue, Bethesda, MD 20814, attn: Special Publishing. Produced in conjunction with the ASHP Publications Production Center.

The information presented herein reflects the opinions of the contributors and reviewers. It should not be interpreted as an official policy of ASHP or as an endorsement of any product.

Drug information and its applications are constantly evolving because of ongoing research and clinical experience and are often subject to professional judgment and interpretation by the practitioner and to the uniqueness of a clinical situation. The editor, authors, and ASHP have made every effort to ensure the accuracy and completeness of the information presented in this book. However, the reader is advised that the publisher, author, contributors, editors, and reviewers cannot be responsible for the continued currency or accuracy of the information, for any errors or omissions, and/or for any consequences arising from the use of the information in the clinical setting.

The reader is cautioned that ASHP makes no representation, guarantee, or warranty, express or implied, that the use of the information contained in this book will prevent problems with insurers and will bear no responsibility or liability for the results or consequences of its use.

Acquisitions Editor: Hal S. Pollard

Editorial Project Manager: Dana A. Battaglia

Project Manager: Johnna Hershey

Page Design: Carol Barrer

Cover Design: Armen Kojoyian

ISBN: 1-58528-052-6

Contents

Chapter 3:

Chapter 4:

Chapter 5:

Chapter 6:

Chapter 7:

Education of Ambulatory Hypertensive Patients 93
Beth Bryles Phillips

Chapter 8:

Ongoing Evaluation and Management of the Ambulatory Patient with Hypertension 113
Tina M. Hisel, Jacqueline D. Joss

Chapter 9:

Referral to Other Health Care Providers 129
Alan H. Mutnick

Chapter 10:

Evaluation of Therapeutic Outcomes 135
Alan H. Mutnick

About This Book

Despite advances in our understanding of the pathophysiology and treatment of hypertension, there still needs to be significant improvements in patient care to further lower the devastating morbidity and mortality associated with this disease. Due to the significant health benefits associated with controlled hypertension and the lack of awareness of the disease, pharmacists have an excellent opportunity to make a positive impact on patient care. Pharmacists can aid in the detection, monitoring, and follow-up of patients with hypertension. They can also help patients meet their blood pressure goals through lifestyle modification and adherence to drug therapy.

Several articles published in the medical literature describe pharmacists in a number of practice settings impacting hypertensive patients in a positive manner. In either independent practice or in collaboration with physicians, pharmacists' interventions have been shown to lower blood pressure, increase the number of patients achieving blood pressure goals, and provide cost-effective management of hypertension.

The purpose of this book is to provide a resource of information for pharmacists and other health care professionals who participate in providing care to patients with hypertension. In addition to providing current and essential information about the treatment and care of hypertensive patients, this book will convey important concepts, knowledge, and advice for patients. Specific aspects of hypertension will be discussed throughout the book, including pathophysiology, measurement of blood pressure, assessment of target organ damage, identification of goals, risk stratification, non-pharmacologic and pharmacologic treatments, development and implementation of a monitoring plan, patient education, referral to other health care providers, and pharmacoeconomics. Each chapter will also include **Clinical Highlights**, a summary of practical information essential for clinicians who are providing care to hypertensive patients and **Key Points for Patients**, a summary of important points for patients. Several cases will be used throughout each chapter to help illustrate key concepts.

Chapter 1:
Introduction to Hypertension

Beth Bryles Phillips

Clinical Highlights

Overview of Hypertension

- Awareness
- Classification
- Causes
- Racial and Ethnic Differences
- Gender and Age-Related Differences
- Target Organ Damage

Summary

References

Clinical Highlights

- How is the most common form of hypertension diagnosed?
- What are some of the risk factors for hypertension?
- What is target organ damage and how can the risk of it be reduced?

Overview of Hypertension

Hypertension is a common and serious disorder affecting approximately 43 million people in the United States, or almost one-quarter of the adult population.[1] It is now the second most common indication for a physician office visit in the United States.[2] Patients with hypertension are at an increased risk of cardiovascular and cerebrovascular diseases, chronic renal failure, and retinopathies.[1,3,4] Hypertension was first recognized as a disease process more than 100 years ago.[4] Since that time, advances have been made in understanding and treating the disease, most notably in the last half of the twentieth century.[5–7] Hypertension leads to increased mortality[5] and lowering blood pressure improves survival.[6]

In an effort to improve the recognition and management of hypertension in the United States, the Joint National Committee on Detection, Evaluation, and Treatment of High Blood Pressure was formed in 1975.[8] This group came together to evaluate the available hypertension literature and provide expert opinion. The first consensus recommendations for management of the hypertensive patient were published in 1977.[8] These recommendations are updated every few years. The seventh and most recent report, commonly referred to as JNC 7, was published in 2003.[9] In addition to the JNC guidelines, other international guidelines on the management of hypertension have been published as well. The most recent and well known are the 2003 European Society of Hypertension–European Society of Cardiology guidelines for the management of arterial hypertension.[10]

Awareness

Despite significant progress in the treatment of hypertension, education of health care providers through the publication of consensus recommendations, and the commonality of the disease, hypertension remains a major modifiable risk factor for cardiovascular disease.[7,9] It is still a major cause of morbidity and mortality in the United States, accounting for approximately 10% of deaths.[11] As many as one-third of patients with hypertension are unaware they have the disease.[9] Furthermore, only one-third of patients with hypertension have blood pressure readings within target ranges.[9] Due to the asymptomatic nature of the disease, tremendous efforts have been made to increase the awareness of hypertension in the general population. One such organized effort is Healthy People 2010, a government publication promoting disease prevention objectives.[12] In this publication, hypertension is recognized and addressed specifically. Among the objectives of this effort are to reduce the percentage of adults with hypertension from approximately 24% to 16% and to increase the percentage of patients with controlled blood pressure to 50%.[12]

Patients with hypertension are often asymptomatic, especially in the early stages. Often, the only sign of the disease is an elevated blood pressure reading. Some patients may have complaints of headache or fatigue but these symptoms are not specific to hypertension. Because patients with hypertension often do not feel *ill*, individuals may have the disease for years before being detected, especially if they do not see a physician on a regular basis. The awareness, treatment, and control of hypertension among Americans improved significantly during the last quarter of the twentieth century[3,6] (**Table 1-1**). These advances in the treatment and control of hypertension lead to dramatic reductions in mortality from stroke and coronary artery disease[13] (**Figures 1-1 and 1-2**). However, the decline in cerebrovascular and cardiovascular mortality has reached a plateau.[13] During the past 10 to 15 years, the age-adjusted rates of stroke incidence and death rate from hypertension have risen and the age-adjusted rate of decline in coronary heart disease has leveled off.[1,11] This is thought to be related to the recent lack of improvement in the rates of awareness, treatment, and control of high blood pressure.[13]

Classification

The seventh report of the Joint National Committee on Prevention, Detection, Evaluation, and Treatment of High Blood Pressure (JNC 7) defines a systolic and diastolic blood pressure less than 120 and 80 mm Hg, respectively, as normal[9] (**Table 1-2**). Blood pressure can be classified into three groups, depending on the systolic or diastolic blood pressure measurement. These groups include stage 1 hypertension, stage 2 hypertension, or prehypertension. In past JNC guidelines, patients with significantly elevated blood pressure could be classified as having a hypertensive urgency or emergency. These patients are now categorized under stage 2 hypertension and decisions for further evaluation, including hospitalization, are based on the presence or absence of other findings suggestive of acute target organ damage.[9] Another common term is *isolated systolic hypertension*, which refers to systolic blood pressure (SBP) greater than 140 mm Hg and diastolic blood pressure (DBP) less than 90 mm Hg. The current JNC guidelines do not make this distinction.[9] Due to cumulative evidence, SBP is recognized as an important cardiovascular risk factor for patients over the age of 50.[14–16]

The 2003 European Society of Hypertension–European Society of Cardiology guidelines utilizes a classification of blood pressure that is similar to previous JNC guidelines (**Table 1-3**). Blood pressure greater than 140/90 mm Hg can be classified as normal; high normal; grade 1, grade 2, or grade 3 hypertension; or isolated systolic hypertension.[10]

Causes

Hypertension can generally be categorized into two groups: primary or essential and secondary hypertension. *Primary hypertension* is a disorder of unknown etiology. It is the most common form of hypertension, characterizing more than 90% of patients with the disease. It is typically diagnosed by the absence of an underlying cause, such as renovascular disease, renal failure, pheochromocytoma, or aldosteronism (**Table 1-4**). In such cases where an underlying cause has been identified, patients are diagnosed with *secondary hypertension*. The focus of this book will be on the care of ambulatory patients with primary hypertension.

Table 1-1.
Trends in the Awareness, Treatment, and Control of High Blood Pressure in Adults ages 18–74*[9]

	National Health and Nutrition Examination Survey, %			
	II (1976–80)	III (Phase 1 1988–91)	III (Phase 2 1991–94)	1999–2000
Awareness	51	73	68	70
Treatment	31	55	54	59
Control†	10	29	27	34

*High blood pressure is systolic blood pressure (SBP) ≥140 mm Hg or diastolic blood pressure (DBP) ≥90 mm Hg or taking antihypertensive medication.

†SBP < 140 mm Hg and DBP < 90 mm Hg.

(Reprinted with permission from the seventh report of the Joint National Committee on Prevention, Detection, Evaluation, and Treatment of High Blood Pressure. National Heart, Lung, and Blood Institute, National Institutes of Health, May 2003; NIH publication no. 03-5233.)

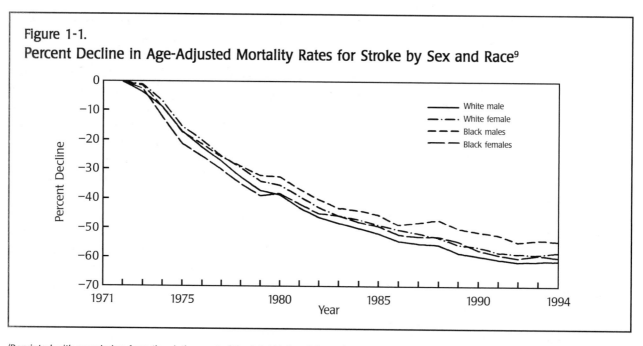

(Reprinted with permission from the sixth report of the Joint National Committee on Prevention, Detection, Evaluation, and Treatment of High Blood Pressure. National Heart, Lung, and Blood Institute, National Institutes of Health, November 1997; NIH publication no. 98-4080.)

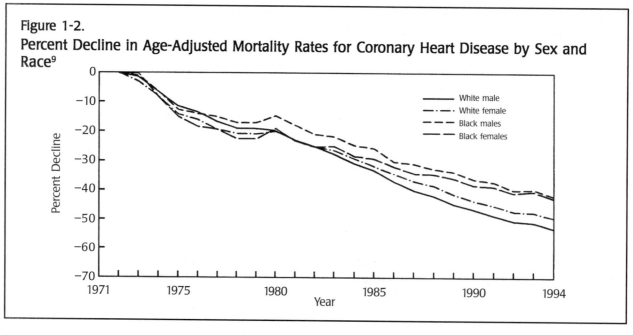

(Reprinted with permission from the sixth report of the Joint National Committee on Prevention, Detection, Evaluation, and Treatment of High Blood Pressure. National Heart, Lung, and Blood Institute, National Institutes of Health, November 1997; NIH publication no. 98-4080.)

Primary hypertension is a result of both genetic and environmental factors.[17] The genetics of hypertension are very complex. There is a definite familial component to hypertension, with a greater contribution from fathers than mothers.[18] Current literature suggests that causes of hypertension are polygenic and related to a number of factors. The development of hypertension itself is dependent upon the interaction of genes with each other as well as environmental factors.[13]

Although little information is currently known about specific genetic variations that cause hyper-

Table 1-2.
Classification and Management of Blood Pressure for Adults*[9]

BP Classification	SBP mm Hg	DBP mm Hg	Lifestyle Modification	Initial Drug Therapy	
				Without Compelling Indication	With Compelling Indications
Normal	<120	and <80	Encourage	No antihypertensive drug indicated.	Drug(s) for compelling indications.[‡]
Prehypertension	120–139	or 80–89	Yes		
Stage 1 hypertension	140–159	or 90–99	Yes	Thiazide-type diuretics for most. May consider ACE I, ARB, BB, CCB, or combination.	Drug(s) for the compelling indications.[‡] Other antihypertensive drugs (diuretics, ACE I, ARB, BB, CCB) as needed.
Stage 2 hypertension	≥160	or ≥100	Yes	Two-drug combination for most[†] (usually thiazide-type diuretic and ACE I or ARB or BB or CCB).	

*Treatment determined by highest BP category.

ACE I = angiotensin-converting-enzyme inhibitor; ARB = angiotensin receptor blocker; BB = beta-blocker; CCB = calcium channel blocker; DBP = diastolic blood pressure; SBP = systolic blood pressure.

[†]Initial combined therapy should be used cautiously in those at risk for orthostatic hypotension.

[‡]Treat patients with chronic kidney disease or diabetes to BP goal of <130/80 mm Hg.

(Reprinted with permission from the seventh report of the Joint National Committee on Prevention, Detection, Evaluation, and Treatment of High Blood Pressure. National Heart, Lung, and Blood Institute, National Institutes of Health, May 2003; NIH publication no. 03-5233.)

Table 1-3.
Definitions and Classification of Blood Pressure Levels (mm Hg)*[10]

Category	Systolic	Diastolic
Optimal	<120	<80
Normal	120–129	80–84
High normal	130–139	85–89
Grade 1 hypertension (mild)	140–159	90–99
Grade 2 hypertension (moderate)	160–179	100–109
Grade 3 hypertension (severe)	≥180	≥110
Isolated systolic hypertension	≥140	<90

*When a patient's systolic and diastolic blood pressure fall into different categories, the higher category should apply. Isolated systolic hypertension can also be graded (grades 1, 2, 3) according to systolic blood pressure values in the ranges indicated, provided diastolic values are <90.

(Reprinted with permission from 2003 European Society of Hypertension–European Society of Cardiology guidelines for the management of arterial hypertension. *J Hypertens.* 2003; 21:1011–53.)

tension, several environmental factors have been identified that increase blood pressure.[1] Some of these factors include obesity, insulin resistance, high alcohol intake, obstructive sleep apnea, excessive salt intake in salt-sensitive patients, aging, stress, and inadequate potassium or calcium intake.[1,19] Many of these factors, such as obesity, can be additive. It is estimated that for each 10% gain in weight, systolic blood pressure may rise by 6.5 mm Hg.[20]

Racial and Ethnic Differences

Roughly one-quarter of the adult population in the United States has hypertension.[11] These percent-

Table 1-4.
Identifiable Causes of Hypertension[9]

Sleep apnea

Drug-induced or related cause

Chronic kidney disease

Primary aldosteronism

Renovascular disease

Chronic steroid therapy and Cushing's syndrome

Pheochromocytoma

Coarctation of the aorta

Thyroid or parathyroid disease

(Reprinted with permission from the seventh report of the Joint National Committee on Prevention, Detection, Evaluation, and Treatment of High Blood Pressure. National Heart, Lung, and Blood Institute, National Institutes of Health, May 2003; NIH publication no. 03-5233.)

ages vary according to age, sex, race, and ethnicity. Groups associated with a higher than average incidence of hypertension include males under the age of 55, African-Americans, people living in the southeastern United States, and people with lower educational and income levels.[1,4,11] Groups associated with a lower than average incidence of hypertension include Caucasians, Asians, Pacific Islanders, and Mexican-Americans.[1,11]

One group that seems to be most affected by hypertension in the United States is the African-American population. They have one of the highest rates of hypertension in the world.[11] Hypertension tends to develop at an earlier age in this population and the average blood pressure tends to be higher when compared to Caucasians. This contributes to a higher rate of target organ damage, such as stroke, coronary heart disease, end-stage renal disease, and death.[11]

Gender and Age-Related Differences

Variations in the rates of hypertension occur between gender and age. Blood pressure (and consequently the occurrence of hypertension) is higher in men than women until the age of 55.[21] The incidence of hypertension after 55 years of age is then higher in women. Blood pressure tends to increase with age, and the incidence of hypertension steadily increases from the second to the sixth decade of life.[1,4] SBP progressively increases with age, while DBP tends to increase until approximately 60 years of age and frequently declines thereafter.[4] Isolated

systolic hypertension is very common in the elderly population and may occur in up to 75% of the hypertensive elderly.[3] These changes are believed to occur due to the lack of arterial elasticity in aging patients.[4]

Target Organ Damage

Sustained hypertension causes damage in a number of different organ systems, including the brain, heart, and kidneys. Patients with hypertension often develop serious complications from their disease, ranging from stroke, myocardial infarction, heart failure, and renal failure. Stroke is probably the most disabling complication of hypertension. However, cardiovascular events and death from cardiovascular causes are in fact far more common.[3]

Compared to normotensive subjects, patients with hypertension have double the risk of experiencing a cardiovascular event and triple the risk of developing heart failure.[3] Hypertension accounts for approximately 35% of all atherosclerotic cardiovascular events.[3] It is also a leading factor in the development of end-stage renal disease and the need for dialysis.[22]

Although patients with elevated blood pressure are at a higher risk for developing cardiovascular complications, treatment of hypertension to control blood pressure does not eliminate the risk for poor outcomes. Rather, overall cardiovascular risk is defined by the level of damage to other organ systems (target organ damage) and specific risk factors[9] (**Table 1-5**). Other cardiovascular risk factors include smoking, dyslipidemia, diabetes mellitus, advanced age, and family history of early cardiovascular disease. Obesity and sedentary lifestyle are also associated with an increased risk of cardiovascular disease.[9]

The presence of preexisting target organ damage, including left ventricular hypertrophy, coronary artery disease, heart failure, stroke or transient ischemic attack, renal disease, peripheral arterial disease, and retinopathy, can also elevate cardiovascular risk in patients with hypertension. Assessing patients for the presence or absence of these risk factors and target organ damage prove important in making treatment decisions and modifying overall patient risk.[9]

One of the most important strategies to reduce the development of target organ damage and cardiovascular complications of hypertension is to

Table 1-5.
Cardiovascular Risk Factors[9]

Major Risk Factors

Hypertension

Cigarette smoking

Obesity (body mass index $\geq$30 kg/m^2)

Physical inactivity

Dyslipidemia*

Diabetes mellitus*

Microalbuminuria or estimated glomerular filtration rate <60 ml/min

Age (older than 55 for men, 65 for women)

Family history of premature cardiovascular disease (men under age 55 or women under age 65)

Target Organ Damage

Heart

- Left ventricular hypertropy
- Angina or prior myocardial infarction
- Prior coronary revascularization
- Heart failure

Brain

- Stroke or transient ischemia attack

Chronic kidney disease

Peripheral arterial disease

Retinopathy

---

*Components of the metabolic syndrome.

(Reprinted with permission from the seventh report of the Joint National Committee on Prevention, Detection, Evaluation, and Treatment of High Blood Pressure. National Heart, Lung, and Blood Institute, National Institutes of Health, May 2003; NIH publication no. 03-5233.)

maintain a goal blood pressure. Although the optimal blood pressure is unknown, the results of several studies have shown that lowering blood pressure can reduce the incidence of cardiovascular events and mortality, cerebrovascular events, and progression of nephropathy.[14,15,23–27] In addition, these benefits have been demonstrated in a variety of special patient populations, including patients with diabetes, isolated systolic hypertension, or no particular coexisting illness.[14,15,23–27]

Summary

Hypertension is a chronic disorder affecting approximately one in four adults in the United States. Because it is an asymptomatic disease in most patients, many people may be unaware that they have the disease. Patients with hypertension are at risk for developing target organ damage, including cardiovascular disease, cerebrovascular disease, chronic renal failure, and retinopathy. Pharmacists have an excellent opportunity to positively impact hypertensive patient outcomes.

References

1. Carretero OA, Oparil S. Essential hypertension. Part I: definition and etiology. *Circulation*. 2000; 101:329–35.

2. Woodwell DA. National ambulatory medical care survey: 1995 summary. Advance data from Vital and Health Statistics; no. 286. Hyattsville, MD: National Center for Health Statistics, 1997.

3. Kannel WB. Blood pressure as a cardiovascular risk factor. *JAMA*. 1996; 275:1571–6.

4. Kaplan NM. Clinical Hypertension. Baltimore: Williams & Wilkins; 1998.

5. Kannel WB, Dawber TR, Kagan A et al. Factor of risk in the development of coronary heart disease—six-year follow-up experience. *Ann Intern Med*. 1961; 55:33–50.

6. Veterans Administration Cooperative Study Group on Antihypertensive Agents. Effects of treatment on morbidity in hypertension. Result in patients with diastolic blood pressures averaging 115 through 129 mm Hg. *JAMA*. 1967; 212:1143–52.

7. Blood Pressure Lowering Treatment Trialists' collaboration. Effects of ACE inhibitors, calcium antagonists, and other blood-pressure-lowering drugs: results of prospectively designed overviews of randomised trials. *Lancet*. 2000; 355:1955–64.

8. Report of the Joint National Committee on Detection, Evaluation, and Treatment of High Blood Pressure: a cooperative study. *JAMA*. 1977; 237:255–61.

9. The seventh report of the Joint National Committee on Prevention, Detection, Evaluation, and Treatment of High Blood Pressure. National Heart, Lung, and Blood Institute, National Institutes of Health, May 2003; NIH publication no. 03-5233.

10. Guideline Committee of the European Society of Hypertension–European Society of Cardiology. 2003 European Society of Hypertension–European Society of Cardiology guidelines for the management of arterial hypertension. *J Hypertens*. 2003; 21:1011–53.

11. American Heart Association. 2002 Heart and Stroke Statistical Update. Dallas, TX: American Heart Association; 2001. http://www.americanheart.org/statistics (accessed 2002 May 24).

12. Healthy People 2010: Understanding and Improving Health. Office of Disease Prevention and Health Promotion, 2001. http://www.healthypeople.gov/document/tableofcontents.htm (accessed 2003 February 7).

13. The sixth report of the Joint National Committee on Prevention, Detection, Evaluation, and Treatment of High Blood Pressure. National Heart, Lung, and Blood Institute, National Institutes of Health, November 1997; NIH publication no. 98-4080.

14. SHEP Cooperative Research Group. Prevention of stroke by antihypertensive drug treatment in older persons with isolated systolic hypertension: final results of the Systolic Hypertension in the Elderly Program (SHEP). *JAMA*. 1991; 265:3255–64.

15. Staessen JA, Fagard R, Thijs L et al. Randomised double-blind comparison of placebo and active treatment for older patients with isolated systolic hypertension. *Lancet*. 1997; 350:757–64.

16. Izzo JL Jr, Levy D, Black HR. Clinical advisory statement: importance of systolic blood pressure in older Americans. *Hypertension*. 2000; 35:1021–4.

17. Harrap SB. Hypertension: genes versus environment. *Lancet*. 1994; 344:169–71.

18. Rebbeck TR, Turner ST, Sing CF. Probability of having hypertension: effects of sex, history of hypertension in parents, and other risk factors. *J Clin Epidemiol*. 1995; 49:727–34.

19. Peppard PE, Young T, Palta M et al. Prospective study of the association between sleep-disordered breathing and hypertension. *N Engl J Med*. 2000; 342:1378–84.

20. Ashley FW Jr, Kannel WB. Relation of weight change to changes in atherogenic traits: the Framingham study. *J Chronic Dis*. 1974; 27:103–14.

21. Burt VL, Whelton P, Roccella EJ et al. Prevalence of hypertension in the US adult population. Results from the Third National Health and Nutrition Examination Survey, 1988–1991. *Hypertension*. 1995b; 25:305–13.

22. U.S. Renal Data System. USRDS 2000 Annual Report. Bethesda, MD, National Institutes of Health, 2000. http://www.usrds.org/atlas (accessed 2001 March 8).

23. Hansson L, Zanchetti A, Carruthers SG et al. Effects of intensive blood-pressure lowering and low-dose aspirin in patients with hypertension: principal results of the Hypertension Optimal Treatment (HOT) randomised trial. *Lancet*. 1998; 351:1755–62.

24. UK Prospective Diabetes Study Group. Tight blood pressure control and the risk of microvascular complications in type 2 diabetes: UKPDS 38. *BMJ*. 1998; 317:703–12.

25. Tuomilehto J, Rastenyte D, Birkenhager WH et al. Effects of calcium-channel blockade in older patients with diabetes and systolic hypertension. Systolic Hypertension in Europe Trial Investigators. *N Engl J Med*. 1999; 340:677–84.

26. Hansson L, Lindholm LH, Ekbom T et al. Randomised trial of old and new antihypertensive drugs in elderly patients: cardiovascular mortality and morbidity the Swedish Trial in Old Patients with Hypertension-2 study. *Lancet*. 1999; 354:1751–6.

27. UK Prospective Diabetes Study Group. Efficacy of atenolol and captopril in reducing risk of macrovascular and microvascular complications in type 2 diabetes: UKPDS 39. *BMJ*. 1998; 317:713–20.

Chapter 2:
Pathophysiology of Hypertension

Jacqueline D. Joss

Clinical Highlights

- Which factors predispose patients to hypertension?
- What presenting features can be clues to the diagnosis of secondary hypertension?
- How does hypertension lead to atherosclerosis?
- Which organ systems are primarily affected as a result of longstanding hypertension?

Pathophysiology of Hypertension

Hypertension is a common contributor to cardiovascular morbidity and mortality. Essential hypertension is the more common form of this disease, and various mechanisms have been proposed to play a role in the pathogenesis. In a small fraction of people, elevation of blood pressure is due to an identifiable cause, which is termed secondary hypertension.

Essential (Primary) Hypertension

The genesis of essential hypertension is multifactorial and complex. In more than 90% of people with high blood pressure, no single cause can be identified.[1] A simplistic explanation of the pathogenesis is that there is an increase in cardiac output, a rise in total peripheral resistance, or a combination of the two, resulting in persistent hypertension. The interplay and the degree of these alterations differ between patients, and this varies with time as compensatory mechanisms interact.[2] The initial changes may occur as a result of changes in the renin-angiotensin system, sympathetic overactivity, or disorders of sodium metabolism.

The kidneys and defects in sodium excretion appear to play a key role in the pathogenesis of essential hypertension.[3] This theory is supported by data from the transplantation literature, in which it was noted that patients who received renal allografts from hypertensive donors were more likely to have higher blood pressure values than recipients who received organs from normotensive donors.[4] Another investigator reported that patients with dialysis-dependent renal failure as a result of longstanding hypertension and without primary renal disease became normotensive when they received kidneys from normotensive donors if the new kidney functioned well.[5] These data (as well as animal data[6]) suggest that hypertension travels with the kidney and that a transplanted kidney which is "genetically programmed for hypertension" will cause hypertension in a normotensive recipient. Some patient groups (e.g., African-Americans and the elderly) have been shown to be sodium sensitive, demonstrating substantial increases in blood pressure as a result of increased sodium intake, also suggesting a renal mechanism of hypertension.[7] Younger patients with hypertension are less likely to demonstrate this syndrome,[8] which supports the theory that other mechanisms are also involved.

Some investigators have hypothesized that essential hypertension often is the result of subtle renal injury.[9] Injury to the kidney may be the result of transient renal vasoconstriction (e.g., as a result of a diet low in potassium or hyperuricemia). Alternatively, a hyperactive sympathetic nervous system may cause transient increases in blood pressure, resulting in renal injury. The resulting ischemia and leukocyte infiltration generate oxidants, which perpetuates the vasoconstriction, resulting in decreased blood flow, capillary injury, decreased sodium filtration, and hypertension.[9]

It has been suggested that a reduced number of nephrons may predispose a person to the development of hypertension.[9,10] This may be caused by an increased susceptibility to injury by transient pressure changes since the lower number of nephrons have hyperfiltering glomeruli.[11] It is unclear whether this reduction in nephrons is caused by genetic or environmental factors. A study in Aboriginal children found an association between low birth weight and low renal volume, which may be an indication of a reduced number of nephrons.[12] Other studies have demonstrated that a change in the intrauterine surroundings have lead to retarded renal grown and decreased birth weight as well as hypertension during adulthood.[13–15]

Other genetic factors have been identified as a cause of inherited hypertension. These are rare and include glucocorticoid-remediable aldosteronism, Liddle's syndrome, mineralocorticoid excess, and autosomal dominant hypertension with bradydactyly.[2,16] Polymorphism of genes involving the renin-angiotensin system, aldosterone synthesis, and adrenergic receptors has been noted to be more common in hypertensive than normotensive people.[17] Genetic changes in the regulation of transport molecules involved in the excretion of sodium may further predispose an individual to become hypertensive.[18]

As discussed in more detail in Chapter 6, environmental factors play a role in precipitating essential hypertension (**Table 2-1**).[1]

High sodium intake will increase fluid volume, which leads to an increase in preload, which in turn will increase the cardiac output. The interactions among potassium, calcium, and hypertension are less well understood. Potassium intake correlates inversely with the prevalence of hypertension. It has been noted that African-Americans ingest less potassium than Caucasians, which may be an explanation for the tendency for more severe hypertension in African-Americans. Hypertension is more prevalent in areas with soft water, which is an indicator that calcium intake is also inversely related to the prevalence of hypertension.

Hypertension has a strong link with obesity and insulin resistance, and it is greater in those patients with central obesity. Obesity and the concomitant resultant hyperinsulinemia stimulate the sympathetic nervous system, thereby contributing to hypertension.[19] This may be the result of a mechanism designed to restore the energy balance and normalize body weight.

Alcohol can have a significant pressor effect when intake exceeds an equivalent of 1 ounce of ethanol per day, which may likely be related to an increase in cardiac output, heart rate, and increased sympathetic nervous system activity. Lack of exercise is linked to hypertension, and it is difficult to determine if this is independent of body fat, since physically fit people usually have less body fat.

Secondary Hypertension (Hypertension with an Identifiable Cause)

Secondary hypertension is defined as elevated blood pressure associated with a specific cause. Secondary hypertension is much less common than primary hypertension; however, it can sometimes be cured when diagnosed and treated with appropriate intervention. **Table 2-2** provides an overview of these disorders and the proposed mechanism by which they cause hypertension.

The kidneys have a pivotal role in hypertension. As discussed earlier, they may predispose to essential or primary hypertension (e.g., reduced number of nephrons). They are also a target for damage as a result of elevated blood pressure. In addition, overt renal disease is also a major contributor to secondary hypertension. Up to 4% of hypertensive patients have concomitant renal diseases.[20] As outlined in Table 2-2, various forms of renal parenchymal pathologies are associated with hypertension. The incidence of hypertension increases even further in terminal renal failure.

Other secondary causes are much less common: primary aldosteronism, Cushing's syndrome, and pheochromocytoma have been noted in 1.5, 0.6, and 0.3% of hypertensive patients, respectively.[21] Due to the relatively low prevalence of secondary hypertension, it has been recommended to only pursue screening for secondary hypertension when certain clinical findings suggest its presence. These include onset of high blood pressure before 20 or after 50 years of age, severe hypertension (e.g.,

Table 2-1.
Environmental Factors in the Pathogenesis of Essential Hypertension

High sodium intake

Low potassium intake

Low calcium intake

Obesity

High alcohol intake

Sedentary lifestyle

Psychological stress

Table 2-2.

Selected Secondary Causes and Mechanisms of Hypertension[1,2]

Diagnosis	Proposed Mechanism of Hypertension	Comments
Renal disease	Salt and water retention, increased plasma volume, and inadequate suppression of renin-angiotensin system may occur.	Of patients with renal parenchymal disease, 20–80% have hypertension. The incidence of hypertension approaches 90% in end-stage renal disease. Examples of parenchymal disease include glomerulonephritis, interstitial nephritis, diabetic nephropathy, polycystic kidney disease, and reflux nephropathy.
Renovascular hypertension	Renin-dependent hypertension, may be secondary to impaired blood flow to the kidneys, often caused by atherosclerosis. Other less common causes include fibromuscular dysplasia, renal artery stenosis, or connective tissue disorders (e.g., Marfan's syndrome).	Incidence may approach 5% of the hypertensive population.
Coarctation of the aorta	Occurs when aorta is narrowed below the origin of the left subclavian artery. Mechanical obstruction and renin-angiotensin activation contribute to hypertension.	Hypertension usually occurs in childhood or early adulthood, and blood pressure is higher in the upper than the lower part of the body.
Pheochromocytoma	Pheochromocytoma cells secrete primarily norepinephine.	This rare condition results from catecholamine-secreting tumors.
Primary aldosteronism[41]	Excess aldosterone production results in potassium loss, sodium retention, and renin suppression.	Rare disorder (0.1% prevalence among unselected hypertensives). Mild forms may be genetic. Various aldosterone-secreting tumors have been described, such as unilateral adrenocortical adenomas (Conn's syndrome), carcinomas, or ectopic tumors in the ovaries.
Cushing's syndrome	Hypertension results from an overproduction of cortisol and a vascular hypersensitivity to angiotensin II and norepinephrine.	Results from increased release of ACTH due to bilateral adrenal hyperplasia. It may also result from tumors producing ACTH-like peptides or from adrenal neoplasms.
Congenital adrenal hyperplasia	Complex errors in the natural pathways and feedback loops result in the accumulation of steroids with potent mineralocorticoid activity.	Genetic errors of corticosteroid biosynthesis are rare causes of hypertension.
Thyroid disease	Atrial natriuretic factor (ANF) is released by thyroid hormones and may therefore be involved in the regulation in blood volume.	Diastolic hypertension occurs in 20% of patients with hypothyroidism. Hyperthyroidism usually results in high systolic pressures.
Pregnancy	Preeclampsia is caused by a marked increase in the sensitivity to vasoconstrictors, resulting in increased peripheral vascular resistance. The underlying cause may be an imbalance in prostaglandins. Blood pressure typically normalizes in the immediate postpartum period.	Preeclampsia usually occurs in nulliparous women in the third trimester of gestation, but it may occur earlier in the pregnancy in women with preexisting hypertension. Proteinuria, edema, and possibly liver function disturbances and microangiopathic hemolytic anemia accompany the disorder. It may progress to eclampsia, which is characterized by life-threatening convulsions.
Obstructive sleep apnea (OSA)	Hypoxia and hypercapnia activate the sympathetic nervous system, thereby elevating the blood pressure during sleep. Hypertension may carry over to the daytime.	Most often occurs in obese patients. Patients have repetitive apneic episodes that result in decreased arterial oxygen content and elevated carbon dioxide levels.
Cardiac surgery	Elevated catecholamine levels and immunosuppressant medications are some of the known contributors to postoperative hypertension.	Transient hypertension may occur after surgery due to pain, physical and emotional stress, hypoxia, hypercapnia, and excessive volume loads. Significant hypertension may develop after coronary bypass surgery, valve replacement surgery, and cardiac transplant surgery.
Iatrogenic hypertension (drug-induced hypertension)	Various mechanisms may be involved: fluid retention, sympathetic stimulation, sodium retention, and increased sensitivity to angiotensin II.	Amphetamines/cocaine, appetite suppressants, cyclosporine, erythropoietin, excessive thyroid hormone replacement, MAO inhibitors (in the setting of tyramine ingestion), nonsteroidal anti-inflammatory agents, oral contraceptives (estrogen), oral decongestants

BP>180/110 mm Hg), or other features that may indicate secondary causes, such as abdominal bruits, variable pressures with tachycardia, sweating and tremor, family history of renal disease, poor response to therapy, or a sudden increase in usually well-controlled blood pressure.[2,22] Clinical features from routine laboratory examinations include unprovoked hypokalemia indicating primary aldosteronism, hypercalcemia relating to hyperparathyroidism, and elevated creatinine levels, which may indicate renal parenchymal disease. As with any clinical assessment, iatrogenic hypertension should be ruled out. This assessment should include a detailed drug history including the use of over-the-counter and herbal medications.

Hypertension as a Risk Factor for Cardiovascular Disease

The vascular complications of hypertension have been classified by some as being either hypertensive or atherosclerotic.[2] The former is caused by the high pressure per se and includes hemorrhagic stroke, congestive heart failure, nephrosclerosis, and aortic dissection. The atherosclerotic complications of hypertension have multiple consequences, as explained later, and include coronary heart disease, arrhythmias, atherothrombotic stroke, and peripheral vascular disease.

The mechanism of hypertension-related consequences, such as atherosclerosis, is complex.[23] It has been suggested that vascular disease is a result of pulsatile flow, endothelial cell dysfunction, and smooth muscle hypertrophy. Hypertension has been shown to have proinflammatory actions, increasing the levels of free radicals. This in turn reduces the formation of nitric oxide and increases peripheral resistance and leucocyte adhesion. These processes mediate some of the effects of hypertension and hypercholesterolemia, which are frequently observed in the same patient. The renin-angiotensin system (RAS) plays a role in the complications of hypertension. Angiotensin II is frequently, although not always, elevated in hypertension, and it can contribute to atherogenesis by stimulating the growth of smooth muscle.[23] Angiotensin II has been shown to activate phospholipase C, leading to increased intracellular calcium, smooth-muscle contraction, and hypertrophy.

Recent data indicate an interaction between the RAS and dyslipidemia.[24] Laboratory studies indicate that elevated lipid levels in the vessels may regulate components of the RAS, while activation of the RAS will stimulate the accumulation of oxidized low-density lipoproteins (LDL). The cross talk between these two systems will increase inflammation and the oxidation of LDL, thus promoting atherosclerosis. This concept suggests that treating hyperlipidemia and blocking the RAS may synergistically improve patient outcome. Further studies are needed evaluating this concept.

Hypertension is currently used as a marker to identify individuals at risk of developing cardiovascular events; however, it is not the ideal marker for identifying the presence of the atherosclerotic complications of this disease.[25] Efforts to develop methods that specifically assess the blood vessels as the site of abnormality are presently not available in clinical practice; therefore, blood pressure remains the surrogate end point at this time. Even though different therapeutic agents may achieve similar levels of blood pressure reductions, the cardiovascular risk reduction is not the same.[26] It has been suggested that systolic blood pressure (SBP) is a better predictor of cardiovascular risk than diastolic blood pressure (DBP), especially in older patients.[27,28] This finding has led to the recommendation by the Joint National Committee on Prevention, Detection, Evaluation, and Treatment of High Blood Pressure (JNC 7) to make SBP the primary focus when treating hypertension.[22] Epidemiological evidence indicates that even though DBP and SBP increase with age, the rise in DBP tends to decrease after the fifth decade of life.[29] In some patients, DBP even decreases after age 50 or 60. These changes may play an important role in myocardial pathophysiology. The increase in SBP increases end-systolic stress, promotes cardiac hypertrophy, and increases myocardial oxygen demand. The lower DBP favors myocardial ischemia, especially in the presence of atherosclerosis in the coronary arteries.[29] This theory has led investigators to believe that pulse pressure (the difference between SBP and DBP) may be a better (and possibly independent) predictor of risk.[29–31]

Target Organ Damage

The consequences of uncontrolled hypertension affect primarily the heart, kidneys, and the brain; however, large vessels such as the aorta may also be affected, resulting in aneurisms and dissections. If hypertension is untreated, 50% of hypertensive patients will die of coronary artery disease or congestive heart failure. About a third of patients with hypertension will die of stroke and up to 15% will develop renal failure. Renal failure is more common in patients with diabetes and in patients with rapidly accelerating hypertension.[1,2]

Cardiac Complications

Left ventricular hypertrophy, coronary artery disease, and congestive heart failure are the principal cardiac complications of hypertension. It has been shown by meta-analysis that controlling blood pressure is the single most effective preventative therapy for congestive heart failure: the efficacy rate exceeded 90%.[32] Hypertension will increase the tension on the left ventricle, which manifests as stiffness and hypertrophy. Hypertension leads to accelerated atherosclerosis, leading to increased oxygen demand and decreased oxygen supply, thereby increasing the likelihood of myocardial ischemia and infarction.

Cerebral Complications

Hypertension is the most important risk factor for spontaneous intracerebral hemorrhage,[33] which may result from ruptured microaneurisms. High-risk patients include those who are noncompliant with antihypertensive medications, smokers, or patients less than 55 years of age.[34,35] Lacunar infarcts can result from thrombotic occlusion of small vessels, and arteriosclerotic disease in the carotid arteries may lead to transient ischemic attacks.[36]

Renal Disease

As already discussed, renal dysfunction may be responsible for the development of hypertension, but it may not be recognized initially. The primary renal complication of hypertension is related to accelerated arteriosclerosis. Mild renal dysfunction, as evidenced by microalbuminuria, has been associated with prehypertensive blood pressure levels of 130–139/85–89 mm Hg.[37] This finding is significant, since microalbuminuria has been found to be a useful indicator for identifying patients at higher cardiovascular risk.[38,39] Chronic renal failure is an uncommon complication of essential hypertension; however, it remains an important cause of end-stage renal disease, especially in African-Americans.[40]

Funduscopic Changes

Retinopathy induced by hypertension is the result of arteriosclerosis. Vascular damage may be progressive, starting with a narrowing of the arteriolar lumen, followed by arteriovenous nicking.[2] Progressive hypertension may cause rupturing of small vessels (hemorrhages and exudates) and papilledema. The latter changes are associated with accelerated-malignant hypertension. Vascular complications in the eye may result in visual changes, including blurred vision, spots, or blindness.

Conclusion

Hypertension is an important risk factor in the incidence of diffuse vascular disease. The mechanisms of disease are complex. The complications of the disease can be decreased by lifestyle modification and medication therapy, which will be discussed in later chapters.

Key Points for Patients

- Rarely hypertension is caused by one identified cause and may potentially be cured. This is termed secondary hypertension. More commonly, however, the cause of hypertension is not fully known (essential hypertension).
- While hypertension is an asymptomatic disease, it can lead to potentially serious complications. The stress on the blood vessels leads to accelerated atherosclerosis. This process leads to diseased (narrowed) vessels in the heart, kidneys, eyes, brain, and other parts of the body. Ultimately these changes can lead to chest pain (angina), heart attacks (myocardial infarction), heart failure, heart rhythm disturbances, transient ischemic attacks, strokes, and kidney failure.

References

1. Waeber B, Brunner H, Burnier M et al. Hypertension. In: Willerson JT, Cohn JN. Cardiovascular medicine. Philadelphia: Churchill Livingstone; 2000:1496.

2. Kaplan NM. Systemic hypertension: mechanisms and diagnosis. In: Heart disease: a textbook of cardiovascular medicine. Braunwald E, Zipes DP, Libby P, eds. Philadelphia: WB Saunders; 2001:941.

3. Cowley AW Jr, Roman RJ. The role of the kidney in hypertension. *JAMA.* 1996; 275:1581–9.

4. Strandgaard S, Hansen U. Hypertension in renal allograft recipients may be conveyed by cadaveric kidneys from donors with subarachnoid hemorrhage. *BMJ* (Clin Res Ed). 1986; 292:1041–4.

5. Curtis JJ, Luke RG, Dustan HP et al. Remission of essential hypertension after renal transplantation. *N Engl J Med.* 1983; 309:1009–15.

6. Rettig R, Folberth C, Strauss H et al. Role of the kidney in primary hypertension: a renal transplantation study in rats. *Am J Physiol.* 1990; 258:F606–11.

7. Weinberger MH. Salt sensitivity of blood pressure in humans. *Hypertension.* 1996; 27:481–90.

8. Midgley JP, Matthew AG, Greenwood CM et al. Effect of reduced sodium on blood pressure: a meta-analysis of randomized controlled trials. *JAMA.* 1996; 275:1590–7.

9. Johnson RJ, Herrera-Acosta J, Schreiner GF et al. Subtle acquired renal injury as a mechanism of salt-sensitive hypertension. *N Engl J Med.* 2002; 346:913–23.

10. Keller G, Zimmer G, Mall G et al. Nephron number in patients with primary hypertension. *N Engl J Med.* 2003; 348:101–8.

11. Kang DH, Nakagawa T, Feng L et al. Nitric oxide modulates vascular disease in the remnant kidney model. *Am J Pathol.* 2002; 161:239–48.

12. Spencer J, Wang Z, Hoy W. Low birth weight and reduced renal volume in Aboriginal children. *Am J Kidney Dis.* 2001; 37:915–20.

13. Barker DJP, Osmond C, Golding J et al. Growth in utero, blood pressure in childhood and adult life, and mortality from cardiovascular disease. *BMJ.* 1989; 289:564–7.

14. Gennser G, Rymark P, Isberg PE. Low birth weight and risk of high blood pressure in adulthood. *BMJ.* 1988; 296:1498–500.

15. Yiu V, Buka S, Zurakowski D et al. Relationship between birthweight and blood pressure in childhood. *Am J Kidney Dis.* 1999; 33:253–60.

16. Carretero OA, Oparil S. Essential hypertension. Part I. Definition and etiology. *Circulation.* 2000; 101:329–35.

17. Sealy JE, Blumenfeld JD, Bell GM et al. On the renal basis for essential hypertension: nephron heterogeneity with discordant renin secretion and sodium excretion causing a hypertensive vasoconstriction-volume relationship. *J Hypertens.* 1988; 6:763–77.

18. Lifton R. Molecular genetics of human blood pressure variation. *Science.* 1996; 272:676–80.

19. Reaven GM, Lithell H, Landsberg L. Hypertension and associated metabolic abnormalities—the role of insulin resistance and the sympathoadrenal system. *N Engl J Med.* 1996; 334:374–81.

20. Brown MA, Whitworth A. Hypertension in human renal disease. *J Hypertens.* 1992; 10:701.

21. Andersen GH Jr, Blakemann N, Streeten DHP. The effect of age on prevalence of secondary forms of hypertension in 4429 consecutively referred patients. *J Hypertens.* 1994; 12:609.

22. The seventh report of the Joint National Committee on Prevention, Detection, Evaluation, and Treatment of High Blood Pressure. The JNC 7 report. *JAMA.* 2003; 289:2560–72.

23. Ross R. Atherosclerosis—an inflammatory disease. *N Engl J Med.* 1999; 340:115–26.

24. Singh BM, Mehta JL. Interactions between the renin-angiotensin system and dyslipidemia. *Arch Intern Med.* 2003; 163:1296–304.

25. Cohn JN. Arteries, myocardium, blood pressure and cardiovascular risk: towards a revised definition of hypertension. *J Hypertens.* 1998; 16:2117.

26. Carter BL. Blood pressure as a surrogate end point for hypertension. *Ann Pharmacother.* 2002; 36:87–92.

27. Kannel WB, Gordon T, Schwartz MJ. Systolic versus diastolic blood pressure and risk of coronary artery disease: Framingham study. *Am J Cardiol.* 1971; 27:335–45.

28. Alli C, Avanzini F, Bettelli G et al. The long-term prognostic significance of repeated blood pressure measurements in the elderly: ten-year follow up. *Arch Intern Med.* 1999; 159:1205–12.

29. Van Bortel LMAB, Struijker HAJ, Safar ME. Pulse pressure, arterial stiffness, and drug treatment of hypertension. *Hypertension.* 2001; 38:914–21.

30. Lakka TA, Salonen R, Kaplan GA et al. Blood pressure and the progression of carotid atherosclerosis in middle-aged men. *Hypertension.* 1999; 34:51–6.

31. Domanski MJ, Davis BR, Pfeffer MA et al. Isolated systolic hypertension: prognostic information provided by pulse pressure. *Hypertension.* 1999; 34:375–80.

32. Moser M, Hebert PR. Prevention of disease progression, left ventricular hypertrophy and congestive heart failure in hypertension treatment trials. *J Am Coll Cardiol.* 1996; 27:1214–8.

33. Brott T, Thalinger K, Hertzberg V. Hypertension as a risk factor for spontaneous intracerebral hemorrhage. *Stroke.* 1986; 17:1078–83.

34. Thrift AG, McNeil JJ, Forbes A et al. Three important subgroups of hypertensive persons at greater risk of intracerebral hemorrhage. *Hypertension.* 1998; 31:1223–9.

35. Qureshi AI, Suri MAK, Safdar K et al. Intracerebral hemorrhage in blacks: risk factors, subtypes, and outcome. *Stroke.* 1997; 28:961–4.

36. Davis BR, Vogt T, Frost PH et al. Risk factors for stroke and type of stroke in persons with isolated systolic hypertension. *Stroke.* 1998; 29:1333.

37. Knight EL, Kramer HM, Curhan GC. High-normal blood pressure and microalbuminuria. *Am J Kidney Dis.* 2003; 41:588–95.

38. Leoncini G, Viazzi F, Parodi D et al. Mild renal dysfunction and subclinical cardiovascular damage in pri-

mary hypertension. *Hypertension.* 2003; 42:14–8.

39. Dell'omo G, Giorgi D, Bi Bello V et al. Blood pressure independent association of microalbuminuria and left ventricular hypertrophy in hypertensive men. *J Intern Med.* 2003; 254:76–84.

40. Klag MJ, Whelton PK, Randall BL et al. End-stage renal disease in African-American and white men. *JAMA.* 1997; 277:1293.

41. Ganguly A. Primary aldosteronism. *N Engl J Med.* 1998; 339:1828–34.

Chapter 3:
Initial Patient Assessment

Alan Mutnick and Tina M. Hisel

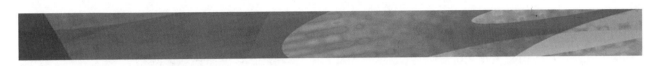

Clinical Highlights

Medical History

Physical Assessment

- Blood Pressure Measurement
- Factors Associated with Inaccurate Blood Pressure Measurements
- Assessment of Target Organ Damage
    - *Funduscopic Examination*
    - *Cardiovascular Examination*
    - *Neurologic Examination*
    - *Examination of Extremities*
- Pulse Pressure and Arterial Stiffness

Laboratory Assessment

- Routine Laboratory Tests
    - *Potassium*
    - *Serum Creatinine*
    - *Urinalysis*
    - *Hematocrit*
    - *Glucose*
    - *Lipoprotein Profile*
    - *Calcium*
    - *Electrocardiogram*

- Optional Laboratory Tests
    - *Microalbumin and 24-hour Urinary Protein*
    - *Uric Acid*

- Laboratory Tests to Rule Out Secondary Causes of Hypertension
    - *Isotopic Renography and Plasma Renin Measurement*
    - *Plasma Aldosterone/Renin Ratio*
    - *24-Hour Urinary Free Cortisol and Dexamethasone Suppression Test*
    - *24-Hour Urine for Catecholamines, Vanilmandelic Acid, and Metanephrines*

Key Points for Patients

References

Clinical Highlights

- What type of assessment should occur during the initial evaluation of ambulatory patients with hypertension?
- How is target organ damage assessed?
- How are the results of a physical examination interpreted?
- How does information obtained from the physical examination help to adequately monitor therapeutic regimens?
- Which laboratory tests should be routinely monitored in patients with hypertension?
- What other laboratory tests may be appropriate when initially evaluating patients with hypertension?
- Which laboratory tests are useful for identifying secondary causes of hypertension?

The initial evaluation of patients with hypertension should include a thorough medical history, physical examination, and laboratory assessment. This diagnostic evaluation allows clinicians the opportunity to screen for secondary causes of hypertension, detect the presence of target organ damage, identify risk factors which may need modification, and develop a treatment plan.

Medical History

Conducting a thorough medical history is essential during the initial evaluation of hypertensive patients. This information will assist clinicians in determining the etiology and guide the diagnostic evaluation. The medical history should include an assessment of:[1]

- Duration and previous levels of blood pressure
- History or current symptoms of target organ damage
- Concurrent cardiovascular risk factors
- Secondary causes of hypertension
- Family history of hypertension, premature coronary heart disease (CHD), stroke, diabetes mellitus, dyslipidemia, or renal disease
- Assessment of lifestyle (e.g., weight gain, physical activity, tobacco use)
- Assessment of diet (e.g., sodium, cholesterol, saturated fat, caffeine, alcohol)

- Prescription, over-the-counter, and herbal therapies
- Illicit drug use
- Previous response and adverse reactions to antihypertensive therapies
- Psychosocial and environmental factors that may influence hypertension control (e.g., family situation, employment status and working conditions, educational level)

Physical Assessment

Physical assessment serves to establish the diagnosis of hypertension and severity of the disease. **Table 3-1** lists the components of the physical examination that should be conducted during the initial evaluation as recommended by the seventh report of the Joint National Committee of Prevention, Detection, Evaluation, and Treatment of High Blood Pressure (JNC 7).[2] This section will describe various components of the physical examination and will provide a stepwise approach to performing certain physical examination skills.

Blood Pressure Measurement

There are many steps involved with blood pressure measurement, and poor technique can result in erroneous measurements. This can lead to inappropriate treatment of hypertension and potential

Table 3-1.

Components of the Physical Examination for Patients with Hypertension[2]

- Appropriate measurement of blood pressure with verification in the contralateral arm
- Examination of the optic fundi
- Calculation of body mass index (BMI)
- Auscultation for carotid, abdominal, and femoral bruits
- Palpation of the thyroid gland
- Thorough examination of the heart and lungs
- Examination of the abdomen for enlarged kidneys, masses, and abnormal aortic pulsation
- Palpation of the lower extremities for edema and pulses
- Neurological assessment

negative outcomes for the patient. This section covers the appropriate technique and factors to consider when measuring blood pressure.

Before blood pressure measurements are obtained, one must be familiar with Korotkoff sounds.[3,4] These represent the various sounds produced by the flow of blood as the constricting blood pressure cuff is gradually released. Five phases of Korotkoff sounds exist. *Phase I* is described as the first appearance of clear tapping sounds and represents systolic blood pressure. *Phase II* represents the change in the tapping sounds to soft murmurs. *Phase III* is represented by louder murmurs as the volume of blood flowing through the constricted artery increases. The sounds become muffled in *Phase IV* when constriction of the brachial artery diminishes as arterial diastolic pressure is approached. All sounds disappear during *Phase V*, which represents the diastolic blood pressure.[5] If the Korotkoff sounds are faint and difficult to hear, the following technique may be useful. Instruct the patient to raise one arm over his or her head and make a fist several times. Inflate the cuff to 50 mm Hg above the expected systolic level while the arm is still overhead but the hand relaxed. Instruct the patient to lower his or her arm rapidly and measure the blood pressure in the usual manner. Draining the venous blood in this fashion often amplifies the Korotkoff sounds and makes weak sounds, particularly diastolic sounds, more audible.

One of the most important steps when measuring blood pressure is to select the appropriate-sized cuff (**Table 3-2**). The bladder within the cuff should cover at least 80% of the midpoint of the bare upper arm. If the cuff is too small or too large, the arterial pressure will be overestimated or underestimated, respec-

tively. A standard cuff is designed for adults with an average-sized arm and measures 5 inches wide. The cuff width should be approximately 1½ inches in infants and small children, 3 inches in young children, and 8 inches in obese adults.[1]

It is essential that the appropriate technique is used when measuring blood pressure to ensure an accurate reading. The patient should be seated in a chair with feet resting on the floor and the arm supported at heart level.[2] Prior to measuring blood pressure, the patient should rest quietly for at least 5 minutes. Two or more measurements should be obtained with verification in the contralateral arm.[2] Minor differences between measurements are common (up to 10 mm Hg). However, differences in systolic pressure exceeding 15 mm Hg might signify obstructive lesions involving the aorta or other major arteries and should be evaluated further. The higher measurement should be used for assessment of blood pressure. **Table 3-3** describes a stepwise approach to obtaining an accurate blood pressure measurement. Problems that may be encountered when measuring blood pressure and recommendations for avoiding these problems are listed in **Table 3-4**.

Patients who experience orthostatic symptoms such as dizziness, lightheadedness, and/or syncope should have their blood pressure measured in different positions. Measuring blood pressure in the sitting or supine position, followed a repeat measurement in the standing position, will help provide evidence of postural changes in blood pressure. A fall in systolic pressure of 20 mm Hg or more, accompanied by symptoms, indicates orthostatic hypotension. This may be the result of antihypertensive medications, loss of blood, or diseases of the autonomic nervous system.

Factors Associated with Inaccurate Blood Pressure Measurements

It is important to recognize that blood pressure measurements may be flawed due to underlying pathology. Pseudohypertension, arrhythmias, and pulsus paradoxus might make it difficult to ascertain the patient's actual blood pressure.

Pseudohypertension is a condition typically found in elderly individuals in which an inappropriately high blood pressure reading is given by sphygmomanometry.[7,8] This is thought to be due to a loss of flexibility of the arterial walls secondary to excessive atherosclerosis. An alternative to

Table 3-2.
Acceptable Bladder Dimensions for Arms of Different Sizes[6]

Cuff	Bladder Width, cm	Bladder Length, cm	Arm Circumference Range at Midpoint, cm*
Newborn	3	6	<6
Infant	5	15	6–15
Child	8	21	16–21
Small adult	10	24	22–26
Adult	13	30	27–34
Large adult	16	38	35–44
Adult thigh	20–42		45–52

*There is some overlapping of the recommended range for arm circumference in order to limit the number of cuffs; it is recommended that the large cuff be used when available.

Table 3-3.
Stepwise Approach to Obtaining an Accurate Blood Pressure Measurement[3]

1. Patients should be seated in a chair with their backs supported and their arms supported at heart level.

2. Blood pressure measurements should not begin until the patient has had at least 5 minutes of rest. Use of tobacco products, ingestion of caffeinated beverages, and exercise should be avoided for at least 30 minutes before measuring the blood pressure.

3. Center the inflatable bladder over the brachial artery. The lower border of the cuff should be approximately 1 inch above the antecubital crease. The cuff should be wrapped snugly around the patient's arm, which should be slightly flexed at the elbow.

4. To estimate the systolic pressure, palpate the brachial artery while inflating the cuff until the brachial pulse disappears. Read the pressure on the manometer and add approximately 30 mm Hg to it. This will provide information on how high to inflate the cuff when measuring blood pressure. Once it has been determined how high to inflate the cuff, rapidly deflate the cuff and wait approximately 30 seconds before measuring blood pressure.

5. Place the bell of the stethoscope over the brachial artery, making sure that an air seal is created with the rim of the bell. Inability to create an air seal will make it more difficult to hear the Korotkoff sounds as they appear.

6. Inflate the cuff rapidly to the predetermined level and slowly deflate the cuff at a rate of about 2–3 mm Hg per second. Deflating the cuff too quickly might result in an inaccurate measurement. The first set of consecutive sounds represents the systolic pressure.

7. Continue to slowly deflate the cuff until the sounds become muffled and then totally disappear. Confirm the total disappearance of sounds by deflating another 10–20 mm Hg, and then deflate the cuff rapidly to zero. The point at which there is a total disappearance of sound represents the diastolic pressure.

8. Record both the systolic and diastolic blood pressures, wait at least 2 minutes, then repeat the measurement.

the use of sphygmomanometry is the measurement of direct intraarterial pressures, which might be necessary in these patients. Several clues might provide evidence of pseudohypertension, including elderly patients with vascular disease, patients who become hypotensive after receiving only modest doses of antihypertensive medications, and patients with elevated blood pressure without evidence of target organ damage.

The Osler maneuver is a technique used to identify patients with pseudohypertension.[7,8] The maneuver is performed by palpating the pulseless radial or brachial artery distal to the point of occlusion by a blood pressure cuff.[9] A patient is considered to be *Osler positive* if the artery remains palpable and *Osler negative* if the artery collapses. One study found that patients who are Osler positive have falsely elevated blood pressure readings compared to true intraarterial pressures.[8] There are conflicting data as to the efficacy of the Osler maneuver. Alternative methods include measuring the patient's blood pressure by way of the fingers. Unlike the larger arteries, which are prone to atherosclerosis, the smaller arteries within the fingers may be more reliable.

Arrhythmias might make it more difficult to adequately determine a patient's blood pressure due to the varying intensity of Korotkoff sounds and error associated with identification at the beginning of regular Korotkoff sounds.

Pulsus paradoxus represents an exaggerated decline in systolic blood pressure of greater than 10 mm Hg with spontaneous inspiration. It can occur in patients with various pathologic conditions, including cardiac tamponade, chronic constrictive

Table 3-4.
Common Problems Encountered When Measuring Blood Pressure[6]

Problem	Result	Recommendation
Stethoscope		
Ear pieces plugged	Poor sound transmission	Clean ear pieces
Ear pieces fit poorly	Distorted sounds	Angle ear pieces forward
Bell or diaphragm cracked	Distorted sounds	Replace equipment
Tubing too long	Distorted sounds	Length from ear pieces to bell should be 12–15 inches
Mercury manometer		
Meniscus not at 0 at rest	Inaccurate reading	Replace or remove mercury
Column not vertical	Inaccurate reading	Place manometer on level surface
Bouncing of mercury with inflation/deflation	Inaccurate reading	Clean tubing and air vent, replace mercury
Aneroid manometer		
Needle not at 0 at rest	Inaccurate reading	Recalibrate
Bladder cuff		
Too narrow for arm	Blood pressure reading too high	Use cuff length 80% of circumference
Too wide for arm	Unable to fit on arm	Use regular but longer cuff
Inflation system		
Faulty valves	Inaccurate reading	Replace equipment
	Difficulty inflating and deflating bladder	Replace equipment
Leaky tubing or bulb	Inaccurate reading	Replace equipment
Observer		
Digit preference	Inaccurate reading	Record to nearest 2 mm Hg
Cut-off bias	Inaccurate reading	Record to nearest 2 mm Hg
Direction bias	Inaccurate reading	Record to nearest 2 mm Hg
Fatigue or poor memory	Inaccurate reading	Write down reading immediately
Subject		
Arm below heart level	Blood pressure reading too high	Place patient with midpoint of upper arm at heart level
Arm above heart level	Blood pressure reading too low	Place patient with midpoint of upper arm at heart level
Back unsupported	Blood pressure reading too high	Avoid isometric exercise during measurement
Legs dangling	Blood pressure reading too high	Avoid isometric exercise during measurement
Arrhythmia	Variable blood pressure readings	Take multiple measurements and average
Large or muscular arm	Blood pressure reading too high	Use appropriate cuff size
Calcified arteries	Blood pressure reading too high	Note presence of positive Osler sign in medical record
Technique		
Cuff		
Wrapped too loosely	Blood pressure reading too high	Wrap more snugly
Applied over clothing	Inaccurate reading	Remove arm from sleeve
Manometer		
Below eye level	Blood pressure reading too low	Place manometer at eye level
Above eye level	Blood pressure reading too high	Place manometer at eye level
Stethoscope		
Applied too firmly	Diastolic reading too low	Place head correctly
Not over artery	Sounds not well heard	Place head over palpated artery
Touching tubing or cuff	Extraneous noise	Place below edge of cuff
Palpatory pressure omitted	Danger of missing auscultatory gap	Routinely check systolic pressure by palpation initially
Inflation level too high	Patient discomfort	Inflate to 30 mm Hg above palpatory blood pressure
Inflation level too low	Underestimation of systolic pressure	Inflate to 30 mm Hg above palpatory blood pressure
Inflation rate too slow	Patient discomfort	Inflate at even rate
Deflation rate too fast	Systolic pressure too low or diastolic pressure too high	Deflate at 2 mm Hg per second or 2 mm Hg per beat
Deflation rate too slow	Forearm congestion	Deflate at 2 mm Hg per second or 2 mm Hg per beat
	Diastolic pressure too high	Completely deflate cuff at end of measurement

pericarditis, emphysema, asthma, hypovolemic shock, pulmonary embolus, pregnancy, and extreme obesity.

Pulsus paradoxus can be detected by inflating the blood pressure cuff to suprasystolic levels followed by a slow deflation of approximately 2 mm Hg per heartbeat. The peak systolic pressure is noted during expiration. The cuff is then deflated even slower, and the blood pressure is again noted when the Korotkoff sounds become audible throughout the respiratory cycle.[4] The normal difference between the two recordings should be approximately 10 mm Hg or less during quiet respiration.

Assessment of Target Organ Damage

As discussed in Chapter 2, hypertension can result in target organ damage such as congestive heart failure, stroke, renal insufficiency, peripheral vascular disease, and retinopathy. The initial physical examination should include an assessment of these specific target organs.

Funduscopic Examination

Hypertension can have deleterious effects on the eyes, including decreased blood flow, appearance of retinal vascular sclerosis, increased arteriolar pressure, appearance of exudates and hemorrhages, and visual defects (e.g., blurred vision, spots, blindness). Vascular changes within the fundus of the eye are reflective of both hypertensive neuroretinopathy and arteriosclerotic retinopathy. A grading system has been developed by Drs. Keith, Barker, and Wagener, which classifies funduscopic changes.[10,11] This grading system is currently referred to as the K-W classification (Table 3-5). Minimizing target organ damage is one of the primary goals of antihypertensive therapy, and the prevention of grades III and IV would be an expected outcome with therapeutic interventions.

The appropriate technique for performing a funduscopic examination with an ophthalmoscope is depicted graphically in Figure 3-1 and described in Table 3-6.

Cardiovascular Examination

A thorough cardiovascular examination should be conducted, including a general inspection; auscultation to identify heart sounds, murmurs, and bruits; and assessment of arterial pulses, jugular venous pressure, and precordial movement.

Under most normal conditions, there are two heart sounds, S1 and S2. However, two additional heart sounds might be heard in patients with hypertension (S4) and in those with heart failure (S3) (Figure 3-2). Auscultation of the carotid arteries is helpful for identifying arterial narrowing, which increases the risk for stroke. The bell of the stethoscope is placed over each carotid artery and the patient is asked to stop breathing for a few seconds. A bruit sounds like a blowing or rushing sound and, if heard, reflects the narrowing of the vessel diameter.

The arterial pulse (heart rate) is typically measured by palpating the radial artery. Measurement of heart rate is routinely performed and can help clinicians identify various rhythm disturbances or blood flow irregularities that would need further evaluation. It can also provide information on the cardiac effects of antihypertensive medications. Table 3-7 describes a stepwise approach to measuring heart rate. The normal heart rate for adults averages between 60 and 100 beats per minute. A heart rate of less than 60 beats per minute is termed *bradycardia* and greater than 100 beats per minute is termed *tachycardia*. The presence of bradycardia or tachycardia is not necessarily an abnormal finding. Bradycardia may be secondary to superior conditioning or parasympathomimetic substances. Patients may experience tachycardia in the setting

Table 3-5.
Keith-Wagener Classification of Funduscopic Changes[10,11]

Level of Involvement	Characteristic Features Found during the Funduscopic Examination
Grade I	Initial narrowing of the arteriolar lumen
Grade II	Sclerosis of the adventitia along with thickening of the arteriolar wall, seen upon examination as arteriovenous (AV) nicking
Grade III	Progressive hypertension results in rupture of the small vessels, which appear as hemorrhages and exudates
Grade IV	Eventual consequence of papilledema

Figure 3-1.
Funduscopic examination.

Looking through the ophthalmoscope, identify the retina. Follow a blood vessel to the optic disk and inspect outward in at least four quadrants. Note any abnormalities.[3]

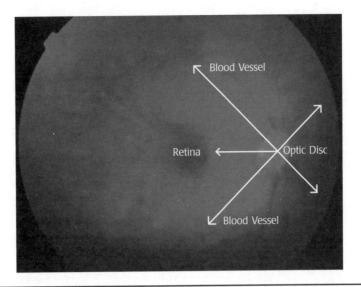

Table 3-6.
Technique for Performing a Funduscopic Examination with an Ophthalmoscope[10,11]

- Adjust the ophthalmoscope so that the light is no brighter than necessary, and adjust the aperture to a plain white circle. The room should be dark.

- Use your left hand and left eye to examine the patient's left eye, and right hand and right eye to examine the patient's right eye. Place your free hand on the patient's shoulder for better control of your movements as you focus on the eye.

- Ask the patient to stare at a point on the wall or corner of the room behind you.

- Look through the ophthalmoscope and shine the light into the patient's eye from approximately 2 feet away. The retina will appear as a "red reflex." Follow the red color and move the ophthalmoscope within a few inches of the patient's eye.

- Adjust the diopter dial to bring the retina into focus; find a blood vessel and follow it to the optic disk. This should be used as your central point of reference.

- Inspect outward from the optic disk and note any abnormalities.

Table 3-7.
Stepwise Approach to Measuring Heart Rate[4]

1. Using the pads of the index and middle fingers, compress the radial artery until you are able to feel maximal pulsation.

2. Note whether the pulse is regular or irregular:
   - Regular beats are evenly spaced, although there might be minor variation with respiration.
   - Regularly irregular beats have a regular pattern but there are "skipped" beats during the measurement.
   - Irregularly irregular beats are chaotic, have no underlying regular cadence, and appear to have no definitive pattern.

3. If the rhythm is regular, count the pulse for 15 seconds then multiply by 4 to estimate the patient's heart rate in beats per minute.

4. If the rate appears to be unusually fast or slow, count the pulse for 60 seconds for a more accurate assessment.

5. Irregular heart rates are difficult to assess by palpating the radial artery. It is generally recommended to use a stethoscope and auscultate the heart directly.

of stress, exertion, cold, sympathomimetic substances, and nervousness.

Jugular venous pressure is inspected to assess right atrial pressure, which if elevated can indicate the presence of heart failure. Jugular venous pressure is reduced upon expiration, but rises in pa-

tients with heart failure (**Figure 3-3**).[3,4] **Table 3-8** lists the appropriate technique for assessing jugular venous pressure.

Observing precordial movements is useful for identifying left ventricular enlargement. The point of maximal impulse (PMI) is produced by left ven-

Figure 3-2.
Auscultation of the heart.

The stethoscope is used to assess cardiac sounds where normally two sounds, S1 and S2, are represented by the traditional "lub dub, lub dub." However, extra heart sounds can also be heard and might reflect pathologic extra sounds in adults due to heart failure-S3 (Figure 3-2a) or hypertension-S4 (Figure 3-2b).[2,3]

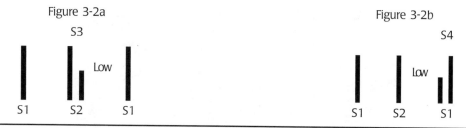

Figure 3-2a

Figure 3-2b

Figure 3-3.
Measurement of jugular venous pressure.

The patient is positioned in a supine position with the head of the table elevated 30 degrees. The first part of the assessment is to identify the highest point of pulsation (Figure 3-3a).The measurement of jugular venous pressure should be less than 4 cm (Figure 3-3b). Increases in the jugular venous pressure occur during cardiac diseases, such as congestive heart failure, due to increases in intracardiac pressures associated with inability of the ventricles to meet the pumping needs of the heart.[2,3]

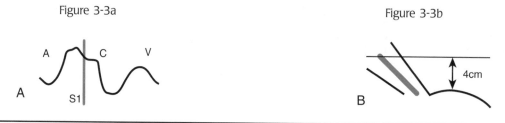

Figure 3-3a

Figure 3-3b

tricular contraction. The normal location of the PMI is medial and superior to the intersection of the left midclavicular line and the fifth intercostal space. The PMI is approximately the size of a quarter and can be displaced in conditions associated with left ventricular enlargement.[3,4]

Neurologic Examination

Hypertension can result in decreased blood flow, oxygen supply, and weakened cerebral blood vessel walls, which may lead to transient ischemic attacks (TIAs), stroke, and the development of aneurysms with potential hemorrhage. These can be accompanied by alterations in mobility, weakness, paralysis, and memory deficits. It is beyond the scope of this chapter to cover all aspects of the neurologic examination, but familiarity with the various parts of the examination are critical in order to effectively monitor patients for signs and symp-

toms of stroke (**Table 3-9**). The use of a Mini-Mental Status Exam (MMSE) may also provide useful information when evaluating the cognitive function of patients who previously suffered a stroke (**Table 3-10**).[12]

Examination of Extremities

The extremities should be examined for edema and pulses. Edema can be the result of congestive heart failure and is typically characterized using a grading system from 1+ to 4+. Hypertension results in occlusive vascular disease of both the proximal and peripheral arteries. Signs and symptoms of vascular disease may include cold extremities, reduced peripheral pulses, and reduced capillary return. **Figure 3-4** depicts the location of various arterial pulses. **Tables 3-11** and **3-12** describe the techniques for evaluating peripheral pulses and capillary return, respectively.

Table 3-8.
Assessment of Jugular Venous Pressure[4]

- Position the patient supine with the head of the table elevated 30 degrees.
- Use tangential, side lighting to observe for venous pulsations in the neck.
- Look for a rapid, double (sometimes triple) wave with each heartbeat. Use light pressure just above the sternal end of the clavicle to eliminate the pulsations and rule out a carotid origin.
- Adjust the angle of table elevation to bring out the venous pulsation.
- Identify the highest point of pulsation. Using a horizontal line from this point, measure vertically from the sternal angle.
- This measurement should be less than 4 cm in a normal healthy adult.

Pulse Pressure and Arterial Stiffness

Current guidelines on the management of hypertension center on the measurement of systolic and diastolic blood pressure, which represent two specific points of the blood pressure wave.[13] Pulse pressure is defined as the difference between systolic and diastolic blood pressure. It has been shown to increase in individuals greater than 50 years of age and may be responsible for the development of accelerated atherosclerosis.[14,15] Several observational studies have provided evidence indicating that pulse pressure is a better predictor of cardiovascular complications in middle-aged and older individuals than mean pressure.[13]

A recent meta-analysis evaluated the role of pulse pressure and mean pressure on the incidence of cardiovascular complications in older hypertensive patients.[13] The authors concluded that the baseline pulse pressure independently predicted the incidence of cardiovascular complications and all-cause mortality when compared to mean pressure. Although the results of this meta-analysis suggest that pulse pressure may be a useful tool for cardiovascular risk assessment, further investigation utilizing randomized controlled trials is still needed.

Arterial stiffness is determined by structural and functional components, which relate to an artery's elastic properties during cardiac pulsation.[16] These elastic properties allow the artery to stretch when pressure is applied and return to its original shape when pressure is removed. Various substances within the intima of an artery are responsible for the degree of elasticity, including elastic fibers, elastin, and collagen.[16] Hypertension has been shown

Table 3-9.
Performing a Limited Neurological Examination[4]

- Observation of facial droop: raise eyebrows, close both eyes, smile, frown, show teeth, etc., in order to assess for weakness, asymmetry, or lag in ability to carry out the task
- Articulation of words (cranial nerves V, VII, X, XII)
- Abnormal eye position (cranial nerves III, IV, VI)
- Abnormal or asymmetrical pupils (cranial nerves II, III), signs of muscle weakness, confusion
- Assessment of motor dysfunction through observation of involuntary movements, atrophy (particularly of the hands, shoulders, and thighs)
- Muscle strength assessment by having the patient move against resistance; flexing of the elbow, extension of the elbow and wrists, squeezing two of your fingers as hard as possible
- Assessment of body reflexes in order to see if there is a central deficit due to stroke. Assessment should include the knees, ankles, biceps, triceps, etc., and should be evaluated bilaterally

to result in elastin degradation and collagen formation.[16] An artery becomes stiffer as the ratio of elastin to collagen decreases. This increase in arterial stiffness results in higher systolic pressures, lower diastolic pressures, and an overall increase in pulse pressure. Arterial stiffness has recently been recognized as an important cardiovascular risk factor and an independent predictor of all-cause mortality and cardiovascular death.[17]

New pharmacologic treatment options are beginning to emerge, which have their primary action on select arterial constituents such as elastin and collagen. One novel drug, ALT-711, works by breaking down collagen bonds and has been shown to decrease the stiffness of blood vessels in elderly people.[18] In one recently published study, ALT-711 altered the properties of the arterial wall, which allowed blood to be ejected more easily from the heart into the peripheral blood vessels. This suggests a potential role of this agent in decreasing arterial stiffness.[18] Ongoing studies with this and other similar pharmacologic therapies will need to be conducted to determine if there is a beneficial effect on cardiovascular morbidity and mortality.

Laboratory Assessment

A baseline laboratory investigation is performed during the initial assessment of hypertensive pa-

Table 3-10.
Folstein Mini-Mental Status Exam[12] (maximum score = 30)

Task	Method for Evaluation	Method for Scoring
Orientation to time	What year is this? What season is this? What month is this? What is today's date? What day of the week is it?	One point for each question answered correctly.
Orientation to place	Which state are we in? Which county are we in? Which city are we in? Which building are we in? Which floor are we on?	One point for each question answered correctly.
Immediate recall	The evaluator names three objects clearly and slowly and asks the patient to repeat the three objects.	One point is given for each object that the patient names correctly.
Attention	Serial 7s: The patient is asked to subtract 7 from 100, then subtract 7 from the answer, and keep subtracting 7 for a total of 5 answers; or have the patient spell the word "world" backwards.	One point is given for each of the serial 7s, which are subtracted correctly; or one point is given for each letter in the word "world," which is spelled correctly.
Delayed recall	Ask the patient to remember the 3 objects mentioned above.	One point is given for each object named correctly.
Naming common objects	Point to two common objects, such as a pencil, pen, or wrist watch, and ask the patient to name them.	One point is given for each of the two objects named correctly.
Repetition	Ask the patient to repeat the following sentence exactly as you say it: "No ifs, ands, or buts."	One point is given if the patient can repeat the sentence exactly as you said it on the first try.
Ability to follow verbal commands	Have the patient listen to the following 3 commands and then have him or her follow your directions: "Take a piece of paper in your right hand, use both hands to fold it in half, and then put it on the floor."	One point is given for each command accurately completed.
Ability to follow written commands	Give the patient a piece of paper that tells him or her to "Close your eyes."	One point is given if the patient closes his or her eyes.
Ability to write	On a piece of paper, ask the patient to write a complete sentence.	One point is given if the sentence has a subject, contains a verb, and makes sense.
Ability to copy an object	Give the patient a sheet of paper and ask him or her to copy a pair of pentagons, which intersect each other.	One point is given if the patient is able to draw an object with 10 corners, which contains 2 intersecting lines.
Scoring	24–30: Within normal limits 18–23: Mild to moderate cognitive impairment 0–17:　Severe cognitive impairment	

Adapted from website located at: http://endeavor.med.nyu.edu/research/pda/pilot/downloads/psychiatry/folstein/folstein.htm.

tients for several reasons. First, it allows clinicians to quickly screen for secondary causes of hypertension. The baseline assessment is also useful for detecting target organ damage and modifiable cardiovascular risk factors. Finally, a biochemical evaluation can be used as a baseline for monitoring the effects of antihypertensive therapy. Table 3-13 reviews the various laboratory tests that may be performed in patients with hypertension.

Routine Laboratory Tests

The basic laboratory investigation should include potassium, serum creatinine, urinalysis, hemat-

Figure 3-4.
Assessment of arterial pulses.

This process involves the complete evaluation of the pulses throughout the entire body, including the toes and feet (tibial and dorsalis pulses), legs (popliteal and femoral), abdomen (abdominal), arms and shoulders (radial up to the brachial), and neck (carotid). Evaluation of pulses is always completed on both sides of the body and characterized as strong or weak. Weak pulses might signify peripheral vascular disease and would warrant further evaluation.

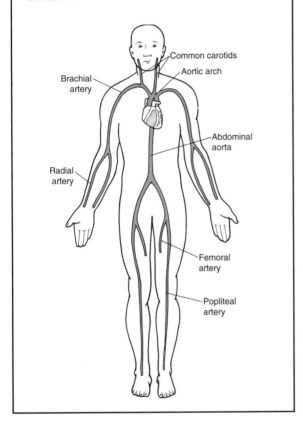

Table 3-11.
Evaluating Peripheral Pulses[4]

- Palpate the radial pulses on both sides of the body. If the radial pulse is absent or weak, palpate the brachial pulses.
- Palpate the posterior tibial and dorsalis pedis pulses on both sides of the body. If these pulses are absent or weak, palpate the popliteal and femoral pulses.
- Weak pulses may indicate occlusive vascular disease and should be noted.

Table 3-12.
Evaluating for Capillary Refill[4]

- Press down firmly on the patient's finger or toenail so it blanches.
- Release the pressure and observe how long it takes the nail bed to "pink" up.
- Capillary refill times greater than 2–3 seconds suggest peripheral vascular disease, arterial blockage, heart failure, or shock.

one secretion.[19] The most serious consequences of altered potassium levels are cardiac arrhythmias, which may ultimately lead to cardiac arrest. The normal range for potassium is 3.5–5.0 mEq/L.[19] Potassium levels less than 2.0 mEq/L or greater than 6.0 mEq/L may result in cardiac arrhythmias and should be treated promptly.

Serum creatinine should be measured at baseline to screen for renal insufficiency. Creatinine is a by-product of muscle metabolism and is eliminated by the kidneys. When renal function declines, the kidneys are unable to filter and excrete creatinine normally, which leads to an increase in serum concentrations. The normal serum concentration ranges from 0.7 mg/dl to 1.3 mg/dl.[19] In general, serum creatinine is normal in the majority of hypertensive patients at baseline. Increases in serum creatinine do not typically occur until more than 50% of renal function is lost.[19]

An assessment of serum creatinine is also necessary when selecting pharmacologic therapy. Several antihypertensive medications can adversely affect renal function or require dose adjustments in the presence of renal insufficiency. Serum creatinine should be reassessed periodically to evaluate the effects of drug therapy and monitor the progression of renal disease.

ocrit, glucose, fasting lipoprotein panel, and electrocardiography.[2]

An assessment of potassium at baseline serves two purposes. First, it allows the clinician to quickly screen for primary aldosteronism. This condition may be suspected if a patient has unprovoked hypokalemia in the setting of hypertension. An evaluation of potassium also provides a baseline for monitoring the effects of antihypertensive therapies (e.g., diuretics, ACE inhibitors, angiotensin II receptor antagonists).

Potassium plays an active role in nerve impulse conduction, muscle cell contractility, and aldoster-

Table 3-13.
Laboratory Tests Used in Evaluating Hypertensive Patients[19,20]

Laboratory Test	Purpose	Normal Range
Blood glucose	• Monitor for diabetes mellitus	<110 mg/dl
Calcium	• Screen for hyperparathyroidism	9–11 mg/dl
Hematocrit	• Identify secondary cause for blood pressure elevation	42–52% (males); 37–47% (females)
Lipid profile	• Identify presence of dyslipidemia	See Table 3-14
Microalbumin	• Used to determine the presence of small amounts of protein in the urine of patients with diabetes mellitus	<30 mcg/mg creatinine during random spot or 24-hour urine collection
Potassium	• Screen for primary aldosteronism • Monitor the effects of certain antihypertensive agents	3.5–5.0 mEq/L
Serum creatinine	• Measure of renal function; screen for renal insufficiency	0.7–1.3 mg/dl
Uric acid	• Monitor effects of certain diuretics • May be a marker for increased risk of cardiovascular events	3.5–8.0 mg/dl
Urinalysis (UA)	• Assess renal function • Identify potential secondary causes of hypertension	Should be free of protein, glucose, red and white blood cells, and casts

Alterations in creatinine should be interpreted with caution because serum concentrations are dependent on body muscle mass. Older individuals tend to have a decrease in their muscle mass and serum creatinine levels might remain in the normal range, despite an age-related decline in renal function. Conversely, muscular patients may have a slightly elevated serum creatinine despite having a normal glomerular filtration rate (GFR). Ingestion of large amounts of meat may also temporarily increase serum creatinine. Creatinine clearance (CrCl) provides an estimation of GFR and is a better assessment of renal function than serum creatinine alone. The Cockcroft and Gault formula is often used to estimate CrCl.[20] It can be calculated using the patient's age, weight, sex, and creatinine in the following formula:

$$CrCl\ (ml/min) = \frac{(140 - age) \times (ideal\ body\ weight\ in\ kg)}{(72 \times serum\ creatinine)} \times 0.85\ for\ women$$

Urinalysis

A urinalysis is performed to assess renal function and identify potential secondary causes of hypertension. Renovascular and parenchymal disorders are the most common causes of secondary hypertension and may be manifested as proteinuria, hematuria, or pyuria.

Urinalysis describes the macroscopic, chemical, and microscopic analysis of a urine sample.[20] The macroscopic analysis consists of a visual observa-

tion of the color and general appearance. A chemical analysis of urine includes pH, specific gravity, protein, glucose, hemoglobin, leukocyte esterase, and nitrite.[20] This can be quickly performed using modern reagent strips, also referred to as dipsticks. Microscopic analysis of urine sediment evaluates the cellular components including white blood cells, red blood cells, epithelial cells, casts, crystals, and infectious organisms.[20]

The urinalysis can detect the presence of proteinuria, hematuria, glucosuria, and casts, which may indicate primary renal disease or nephrosclerosis.[20] Other aspects of the urinalysis are beyond the scope of this discussion and will not be reviewed. The kidneys normally excrete a small amount of protein. The normal range for protein in the urine is 0 to 1+, or less than 150 mg/day.[19] A urine dipstick showing more than 1+ protein should be evaluated further by a 24-hour urine collection to estimate total protein excretion. Glucose is not normally present in urine. If glucose is detected, it could indicate the presence of hyperglycemia. Glucosuria with normal serum glucose concentrations could indicate the presence of renal tubular dysfunction. Hemoglobin is not normally present in urine, and hematuria may be secondary to glomerular lesions.

Ideally, there should not be any cells in the microscopic analysis of urine. However, the presence of a few cells is not uncommon. Excessive numbers of red blood cells (more than 5–10 per high-power field) could indicate the presence of renal disease, infection, kidney stones, or a tumor in the kidneys or urinary system.[20] White blood cells greater than 5–10 per high-power field may indicate pyelonephritis.[20] Casts in the urine sediment help to distinguish the presence of renal disease from urinary system disease. Red blood cell casts are present in proliferative glomerulonephritis. Epithelial cell casts may indicate the presence of acute tubular necrosis, glomerulonephritis, or nephrotic syndrome.

Hematocrit

Hematocrit reflects the percent of whole blood that is occupied by red blood cells. High hematocrit concentrations increase blood viscosity. There is a subsequent increase in blood pressure in an effort to circulate the more viscous blood throughout the vasculature. The JNC 7 guidelines recommend the routine measurement of hematocrit at baseline when evaluating patients with hypertension.[2] The reference range for hematocrit is 42–52% for males and 37–47% for females.[20]

Glucose

Serum glucose should be measured at baseline to screen for diabetes mellitus. Patients with diabetes have an increased incidence of macrovascular complications including cardiovascular, cerebrovascular, and peripheral vascular disease. In addition, diabetic patients are at an increased risk for microvascular complications including nephropathy, retinopathy, and peripheral neuropathy.

Glucose provides most of the energy for cellular and tissue functions and is necessary to sustain life. Glucose enters the body primarily as disaccharides, which are then enzymatically cleaved to monosaccharides for absorption in the intestines. Persistently elevated glucose levels indicate the presence of diabetes mellitus.

According to the American Diabetes Association, diabetes mellitus can be diagnosed three ways: (1) symptoms of diabetes and casual plasma glucose concentration >200 mg/dl; (2) fasting plasma glucose >126 mg/dl; or (3) 2-hour plasma glucose >200 mg/dl during an oral glucose tolerance test.[21] The classic symptoms of diabetes include polyuria, polydipsia, and unexplained weight loss. The fasting plasma glucose method is preferred due to the ease of administration, acceptability to patients, and lower cost. These criteria should be confirmed

by repeat testing on a different day. It should be noted that different criteria are used to diagnose gestational diabetes in pregnant women.

Lipoprotein Profile

A fasting lipoprotein profile should be obtained to detect the presence of dyslipidemia, a major risk factor for cardiovascular disease.[22] Evidence from clinical trials suggests that, for each 1% reduction in serum cholesterol levels, there is an approximate 2% reduction in the rate of fatal and nonfatal coronary artery disease.[23] Therefore, early detection of dyslipidemia is necessary to decrease the risk for cardiovascular disease. Certain antihypertensive medications may also adversely affect lipids (e.g., beta blockers, diuretics); therefore, a baseline assessment will allow clinicians to monitor the effects of therapy.

A lipoprotein profile consists of total cholesterol, low-density lipoprotein (LDL) cholesterol, high-density lipoprotein (HDL) cholesterol, and triglycerides. Cholesterol is a fatlike substance that travels in the body as lipoproteins, which include LDL, very-low-density lipoproteins (VLDL), and HDL. Most of the serum cholesterol is contained in LDL, which is the major atherogenic lipoprotein. Total cholesterol is a measure of all of the lipoproteins in the blood, and the concentration of total cholesterol is correlated with LDL cholesterol. Recent data have implicated elevated triglycerides as an independent risk factor for coronary artery disease.[22] HDL cholesterol acts as a protective lipoprotein against atherogenesis. Studies have demonstrated that low HDL cholesterol levels increase the risk for coronary heart disease, which is independent of LDL cholesterol and other risk factors. The classification of lipoproteins is summarized in **Table 3-14.**

Calcium

Serum calcium should be measured to screen for hyperparathyroidism. The parathyroid glands release parathyroid hormone (PTH) in response to low serum calcium levels. This results in calcium mobilization from bones and increased urinary calcium retention, which returns calcium levels to normal. Hyperparathyroidism results in hypercalcemia, and individuals with this disorder often have hypertension.[24] The reference range for calcium is 9–11 mg/dl.[19] When interpreting serum calcium levels, it is important to evaluate albumin concen-

Table 3-14.
Classification of Lipoproteins (mg/dl)[22]

LDL cholesterol

<100	Optimal
100–129	Near or above optimal
130–159	Borderline high
160–189	High
>190	Very high

Total cholesterol

<200	Desirable
200–239	Borderline high
>240	High

HDL cholesterol

<40	Low
>60	High

Triglycerides

<150	Normal
150–199	Borderline high
200–499	High
>500	Very high

trations as well because 0.8 mg of calcium is bound to 1.0 g of albumin in the serum.[19]

Electrocardiogram

An electrocardiogram (ECG) measures the electrical activity of the heart and provides information about target organ damage.[25] Myocardial ischemia is characterized by inverted T waves, and the presence of Q waves indicates myocardial infarction.[25] ST segment elevation indicates an acute or recent infarction. An ECG can also detect the presence of left ventricular hypertrophy (LVH), which increases the risk for cardiovascular events. LVH can be detected on an ECG by the presence of inverted and asymmetrical T waves.[25] LVH can also be determined by measuring the depth of the S wave in V_1 and the height of the R wave in V_5. If these measure more than 35 mm when added together, this indicates LVH.[25]

Optional Laboratory Tests

Optional laboratory tests may be useful in some patients based on the information gathered from the history and physical examination. These include microalbumin, 24-hour urinary protein, and uric acid.

Microalbumin and 24-hour Urinary Protein

If initial screening tests indicate the presence of diabetes mellitus or initial urinalysis is positive for protein, an assessment of microalbumin is warranted. Microalbumin can be quantitatively measured using three different methods: random spot collection, timed collection, and 24-hour urine collection.

Criteria for the diagnosis of microalbuminuria and clinical albuminuria are shown in **Table 3-15**. Positive tests should be repeated due to day-to-day variability in urinary albumin excretion. It is recommended that two out of three tests are positive in a 3–6-month time period before the diagnosis of microalbuminuria is made.[21]

Uric Acid

Uric acid levels may be elevated in patients with hypertension secondary to decreased renal function. Available data suggest hyperuricemia is associated with an increased risk of cardiovascular events. It is suggested that serum uric acid levels be measured in patients at risk for cardiovascular disease as it carries prognostic information. Diuretic use may also cause hyperuricemia, with thiazide diuretics resulting in elevated uric acid levels more often than other types of diuretics. Diuretic-induced hyperuricemia may precipitate gout attacks in predisposed individuals. Normal uric acid levels range from 3.5 to 8.0 mg/dl.[19]

Laboratory Tests to Rule Out Secondary Causes of Hypertension

A secondary cause of hypertension may be suspected in patients who have an abrupt onset of hypertension, those with severe hypertension (>180/110 mm Hg), or those who have hypertension that is difficult to control despite maximal medical therapy. A more extensive laboratory evaluation may be necessary if a secondary cause of hypertension is suspected. The most common secondary causes of hypertension are renovascular disease, primary aldosteronism, Cushing's syndrome, and pheochromocytoma. This section briefly describes laboratory tests used in the screening of these disorders. Reference ranges for the following laboratory tests can be found in **Table 3-16**.

Table 3-15.
Diagnosis of Microalbuminuria and Clinical Albuminuria[21]

	Random Spot Collection, mcg/mg creatinine	Timed Collection, mcg/min	24-hour Collection, mg/24 hours
Microalbumin	30–299	20–199	30–299
Albuminuria	>300	>200	>300

Table 3-16.
Laboratory Tests to Evaluate Secondary Causes of Hypertension[19,20]

Laboratory Test	Diagnostic Criteria	Comments
Renovascular hypertension Plasma renin measurement	• Stimulated plasma renin >12 ng/ml/hr • Absolute increase of 10 ng/ml/hr • At least 1.5 to 4-fold increase in plasma renin from baseline	• Patients must discontinue diuretics and ACE inhibitors, and consume a normal sodium diet. • Definitive tests include renal arteriography and renal-vein renin determinations.
Primary hyperaldosteronism Plasma aldosterone to renin ratio	• Ratio >20	• No specific preparation or conditions are necessary to perform this test. • Confirmation of this disorder requires measurement of aldosterone excretion via a 24-hour urine collection.
Cushing's syndrome 24-Hour urinary free cortisol level	• >100 mcg/24 hours	• Abnormal screening test results should be evaluated further with additional tests.
Plasma cortisol level	• >7 mcg/100 mg	• Abnormal screening test results should be evaluated further with additional tests.
Pheochromocytoma 24-Hour urinary epinephrine level	• >20 mcg	• Abnormal screening test results should be confirmed using other methods.
24-Hour urinary norepinephrine level	• >100 mcg	• Abnormal screening test results should be confirmed using other methods.
24-Hour urinary metanephrine and normetanephrine level	• >1.3 mg	• Abnormal screening test results should be confirmed using other methods.
24-Hour urinary VMA level	• >6 mg	• Abnormal screening test results should be confirmed using other methods.

Isotopic Renography and Plasma Renin Measurement

The initial screening tests for the diagnosis of renovascular hypertension are plasma renin measurement after an oral captopril challenge and isotopic renography.[20] This disorder should be suspected as a cause for hypertension if the patient's blood pressure is hard to control, if the hypertension is associated with worsening renal function, or if the increase in blood pressure is of new onset.

The use of the laboratory for the diagnosis of renovascular disease is aimed at documenting high levels of renin. Plasma renin and isotopic flow are measured 1 hour after the administration of a single 50-mg dose of captopril. Isotopic renography uses labeled hippurate to measure renal blood flow and DTPA or MAG 3 to measure the glomerular filtration rate.

Plasma Aldosterone/Renin Ratio

Plasma aldosterone/renin ratio is the screening test used in the diagnosis of primary hyperaldosteronism.[20] This diagnosis should be considered when hypertension and low serum potassium (<3.5 mEq/L) occur simultaneously. It is estimated that patients with these characteristics have primary hyperaldosteronism 50% of the time. This disorder is the result of adrenal hyperfunction, which is most often due to a solitary benign adenoma. Adrenal hyperfunction results in excessive aldosterone secretion, which subsequently suppresses plasma renin activity. Aldosterone excess can increase blood pressure and cause hypokalemia.

24-Hour Urinary Free Cortisol and Dexamethasone Suppression Test

A 24-hour urinary free cortisol measurement and overnight dexamethasone suppression test are screening tests used in the diagnosis of Cushing's syndrome.[20] Patients with Cushing's syndrome produce an excessive amount of ACTH, which results in glucocorticoid and mineralocorticoid excess. ACTH stimulates aldosterone production. As a result, patients with this disorder often have hypertension. To perform this test, a 24-hour urine is obtained and the free cortisol level is measured. For the dexamethasone suppression test, 1 mg of dexamethasone is administered at bedtime. A plasma cortisol level is drawn between 7:00 and 10:00 a.m.

24-Hour Urine for Catecholamines, Vanilmandelic Acid, and Metanephrines

The 24-hour urine assay for catecholamines, vanillylmandelic acid (VMA), and metanephrines is the best screening procedure for pheochromocytoma, a tumor arising from chromaffin cells of the sympathetic nervous system.[19,20] This rare condition occurs in 0.1–0.2% of the hypertensive population.[19] These tumors secrete epinephrine, norepinephrine, and dopamine. This can result in sustained hypertension in approximately 50% of the patients, or paroxysmal episodes of hypertension.

Approximately 3–6% of epinephrine and norepinephrine are excreted unchanged by the kidneys. The remainder is metabolized to VMA and metanephrines. These substances can be measured in the urine while the patient is hypertensive to aid in the diagnosis of pheochromocytoma. There are several factors that may increase the production of catecholamines, including certain foods, medications, and stress. Therefore, abnormal screening tests should be confirmed using other methods.

Key Points for Patients

- Prevention, detection, and treatment of hypertension require continuous monitoring for improvement in order to minimize the long-term complications associated with it.
- The goal of antihypertensive treatment is to reduce morbidity and mortality from cardiovascular, neurologic, renal, retinal, and peripheral vascular diseases associated with uncontrolled blood pressure.
- The accuracy of blood pressure readings depends on proper technique as well as the conditions under which the measurements are being made. Blood pressure measurements taken at home can help provide a more complete picture of the patient's blood pressure control but need to be carried out accurately.
- Laboratory tests help detect any damage that has been done to the body due to high blood pressure.
- Laboratory tests assist health care providers with identifying disease states that may increase blood pressure and are also useful for identifying risk factors for cardiovascular disease.
- Certain antihypertensive medications may adversely affect laboratory tests. Therefore, it is important to monitor these laboratory tests periodically.

References

1. The sixth report of the Joint National Committee on Prevention, Detection, Evaluation, and Treatment of High Blood Pressure. *Arch Intern Med.* 1997; 157:2413–46.

2. The seventh report of the Joint National Committee on Prevention, Detection, Evaluation, and Treatment of High Blood Pressure. The JNC 7 report. *JAMA.* 2003; 289:2560–72.

3. Bickley LS, Hoekelman RA, eds. Bates guide to physical examination and history taking, 7th ed. Philadelphia: Lippincott Williams & Wilkins; 1998.

4. Rathe R, MD. University of Florida, 1998. http://www.medinfo.ufl.edu/year1/bcs/clist/index.html (accessed 2003 Apr 15).

5. Franklin SS, Khan SA, Wong ND et al. Is pulse pressure useful in predicting risk for coronary heart disease? The Framingham heart study. *Circulation.* 1999; 100:354–60.

6. Perloff D, Grim C, Flack J et al. Human blood pressure determination by sphygmomanometry. *Circulation.* 1993; 88:2460–7.

7. Chae CU, Pfeffer MA, Glynn RJ et al. Increased pulse pressure and risk of heart failure in the elderly. *JAMA.* 1999; 281:634–9.

8. Messerli FH, Ventura HO, Amodeo C. Osler's maneuver and pseudohypertension. *N Engl J Med.* 1985; 312:1548–51.

9. Cheng TO. Osler maneuver to detect pseudohypertension. *JAMA.* 1999; 282(10):943.

10. Lip GYH. University Department of Medicine, City Hospital, Birmingham, England http://www.fac.org.ar/scvc/llave/hbp/lip/sld004.htm (accessed 2003 Apr 15).

11. The Medical Algorithm Project, Released October 2002. http://www.medal.org/docs_ch19/doc_ch19.08.html (accessed 2003 Apr 15).

12. Chou J. University of Nevada, School of Medicine. Folstein's Mini-Mental Status Download Page website address: http://endeavor.med.nyu.edu/research/pda/pilot/downloads/psychiatry/folstein/folstein.htm, accessed on January 29, 2004.

13. Blacher J, Staessen JA, Girerd X et al. Pulse pressure not mean pressure determines cardiovascular risk in older hypertensive patients. *Arch Intern Med.* 2000; 160:1085–9.

14. Franklin SS, Gustin W, Wong ND et al. Hemodynamic patterns of age related changes in blood pressure. The Framingham study. *Circulation.* 1997; 96:308–15.

15. Kristjansson K, Sigurdsson JA, Lissner L et al. Blood pressure and pulse pressure development in a population sample of women with special reference to basal body mass and distribution of body fat and their changes during 24 years. *Int J Obes.* 2003; 27:128–33.

16. Arnett DK. Arterial stiffness and hypertension. http://www.fac.org.ar/scvc/llave/PDF/arnetti.PDF (accessed 2003 Apr 21).

17. Mahmud A, Feely J. Effect of smoking on arterial stiffness and pulse pressure amplification. *Hypertension.* 2003; 41:183–7.

18. Kass DA, Shapiro EP, Kawaguchi M et al. Improved arterial compliance by a novel advanced glycation end-product crosslink breaker. *Circulation.* 2001; 104:1464–70.

19. Wallach J. Interpretation of diagnostic tests, 7th ed. Philadelphia: Lippincott Williams & Wilkins; 2000.

20. Sacher RA, McPherson RA. Widmann's clinical interpretation of laboratory tests, 10th ed. Philadelphia: FA Davis; 1991.

21. The Expert Committee on the Diagnosis and Classification of Diabetes Mellitus. American Diabetes Association: Clinical practice recommendations 2003. *Diabetes Care.* 2003; 26:S1–156.

22. Expert Panel on Detection, Evaluation, and Treatment of High Blood Cholesterol in Adults. Executive summary of the third report of the National Cholesterol Education Program (NCEP) Expert Panel on Detection, Evaluation, and Treatment of High Blood Cholesterol in Adults (Adult Treatment Panel III).

23. Johnson CL, Rifkind BM, Sempos CT et al. Declining serum total cholesterol levels among US adults. *JAMA.* 1993; 269:3002–8.

24. Lafferty FW. Primary hyperparathyroidism. Changing clinical spectrum, prevalence of hypertension, and discriminant analysis of laboratory tests. *Arch Intern Med.* 1981; 141:1761–6.

25. Dubin D. Rapid interpretation of EKG's, 4th ed. Tampa: Cover Inc.; 1989.

Chapter 4:
Identification of Treatment Goals

Tina M. Hisel

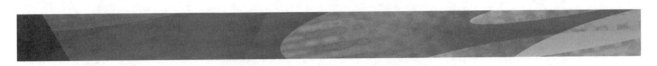

Clinical Highlights

Identification of Cardiovascular Risk Factors

- Cigarette Smoking
- Dyslipidemia
- Diabetes Mellitus
- Age
- Family History of Premature CHD
- Obesity
- Abdominal Obesity
- Physical Inactivity
- Psychosocial Factors
- Ethnic Characteristics
- Small, Dense LDL
- Lipoprotein(a)
- Fibrinogen
- C-Reactive Protein
- Homocysteine

Goals of Treatment

- Blood Pressure Control
- Risk Factor Modification
- Antiplatelet Therapy

Patient Involvement When Establishing Treatment Goals

Key Points for Patients

Patient Case

References

Clinical Highlights

- What are the cardiovascular risk factors to consider when establishing treatment goals for patients with hypertension?
- What are the blood pressure goals for hypertensive patients?
- What are the goals for patients with concurrent cardiovascular risk factors?
- What role does aspirin play in the evaluation and treatment of patients with hypertension?
- Why is it important to involve patients when establishing treatment goals?

An important step during the initial assessment of patients with hypertension includes establishment of treatment goals. Identification of common and individual goals for patients not only helps to guide treatment decisions but will also involve patients in their health care.

When establishing treatment goals, it is necessary to take into consideration not only the level of blood pressure but also the overall cardiovascular risk. This can be accomplished by evaluating the presence of cardiovascular risk factors, target organ damage, and clinical cardiovascular disease. Utilizing the information collected during the medical history, physical examination, and laboratory assessment can assist the clinician with establishing treatment goals.

Identification of Cardiovascular Risk Factors

In addition to hypertension, there are several other risk factors that contribute to coronary heart disease (CHD) risk. Major risk factors have been shown to have a strong, graded, and independent relationship with CHD risk.[1] Other cardiovascular risk factors (predisposing and conditional) have also been identified; however, their independent contribution to CHD risk is not as clear.[2] Government agencies and professional societies generally agree on several major cardiovascular risk factors, but there are some differences in the classification

of independent risk factors for CHD.[2–6] **Table 4-1** lists independent risk factors for CHD by professional society or government agency. All pertinent risk factors will be discussed briefly to give the reader a better understanding of how they contribute to overall CHD risk.

Cigarette Smoking

Cigarette smoking increases the risk for fatal CHD by 70% and imparts a 2–4-fold increased risk of nonfatal CHD and sudden death.[7] In addition, it causes or contributes to many other adverse health outcomes such as cancer, lung disease, and osteoporosis. It is one of the most important modifiable risk factors. Acutely, cigarette smoking results in uninhibited platelet aggregation and sympathetic nervous system stimulation.[8] These effects can result in myocardial infarction, stroke, and sudden death. Chronic use of cigarettes increases the formation of atherosclerotic plaques with long-term consequences.[8] This is due to alterations in lipid concentrations [i.e., decreased high-density lipoproteins (HDL), increased low-density lipoproteins (LDL), and increased triglycerides], increased fibrinogen and factor VII, decreased plasminogen, increased plasma viscosity, and endothelial damage.[8]

Dyslipidemia

Research has shown that altered cholesterol levels, in particular elevated LDL cholesterol, increases the risk for CHD.[6] The National Cholesterol Education

Table 4-1.
Major Independent Risk Factors for CHD[11]

Risk Factor	ACC[2]	AHA[3]	JNC 7[4]	ESH–ESC	ATP III[6]
Cigarette smoking	X	X	X	X	X
Elevated blood pressure	X	X	X	X	X
Dyslipidemia	X	X	X	X	X
Diabetes mellitus	X	X	X	X	X
Age	X	X	X	X	X
			(Men >55 yr)	(Men >55 yr)	(Men ≥45yr)
			(Women >65 yr)	(Women >65 yr)	(Women ≥55 yr)
Family history of premature CHD			X	X	X
			(Men <55 yr)		
			(Women <65 yr)		
Physical inactivity		X	X		
Obesity (including abdominal obesity)		X	X		
Microalbuminuria or estimated GFR <60 ml/min			X		

ACC = American College of Cardiology

*AHA = American Heart Association

JNC 7 = The seventh report of the Joint National Committee on Prevention, Detection, Evaluation, and Treatment of High Blood Pressure

ESH–ESC = 2003 European Society of Hypertension–European Society of Cardiology Guidelines for the Management of Arterial Hypertension

ATP III = National Cholesterol Education Program (NCEP) Expert Panel on Detection, Evaluation, and Treatment of High Blood Cholesterol in Adults (Adult Treatment Panel III).

Program's Adult Treatment Panel III (ATP III) guidelines now identify elevated LDL cholesterol as the primary target when treating dyslipidemia and has placed less emphasis on total cholesterol.[6] Low HDL cholesterol has also been found to be a major risk factor for CHD; however, it is not the primary target for treatment.[6]

Historically, the role of elevated triglycerides on CHD risk has been conflicting. Based on a recent meta-analysis of prospective studies, the ATP III guidelines now recognize elevated triglycerides as an independent risk factor for CHD.[6,9] In patients with high triglycerides (≥200 mg/dl), ATP III identifies non-HDL cholesterol (defined as total cholesterol minus HDL cholesterol) as the secondary target.[6] Non-HDL cholesterol goals are 30 mg/dl higher than LDL cholesterol goals. ATP III does not define a goal for increasing HDL cholesterol due to insufficient evidence from clinical trials.[6] Table 4-2 classifies cholesterol according to the ATP III guidelines. The reader should refer to the guidelines for further information on estimating 10-year risk for men and women with dyslipidemia.[6]

Table 4-2.
Classification of Cholesterol (mg/dl)[6]

Cholesterol	Classification
LDL cholesterol	
<100	Optimal
100–129	Near or above optimal
130–159	Borderline high
160–189	High
≥190	Very high
Total cholesterol	
<200	Desirable
200–239	Borderline high
≥240	High
HDL cholesterol	
<40	Low
≥60	High
Serum triglycerides	
<150	Normal
150–199	Borderline high
200–499	High
≥500	Very high

Diabetes Mellitus

Diabetes mellitus is associated with significant morbidity and mortality. Patients with diabetes are predisposed to atherosclerosis and have a 2 to 4-fold increased risk of CHD.[10] Their cardiovascular risk profile is similar to those patients with established CHD.[11] As a result, diabetes is often considered a CHD risk equivalent. Individuals with diabetes tend to have several other risk factors for cardiovascular disease, including hypertension, dyslipidemia, and obesity. It has been estimated that patients with diabetes and hypertension have twice the risk of CHD than nondiabetic patients with hypertension.[10]

Age

The risk for CHD increases continuously with age, and available data demonstrate higher CHD rates in the elderly. This is likely due to atherosclerotic changes with age.[2] The age criteria vary among authorities as indicated in Table 4-1.

Family History of Premature CHD

A positive family history of premature CHD increases an individual's risk of CHD as demonstrated in the Framingham Heart Study.[12] The ATP III guidelines define premature CHD as a definite myocardial infarction or sudden death before age 55 in a male first-degree relative, or before age 65 in a female first-degree relative.[6]

Obesity

Obesity is the second leading cause of preventable death in the United States and is associated with an increased all-cause mortality.[13] Approximately 55% of Americans over the age of 20 are overweight or obese.[13] Body mass index (BMI) is the accepted measure of an individual's weight status and is the most desirable measure of obesity. BMI can be calculated by taking the patient's weight in kilograms divided by his or her height in meters squared (kg/m^2). Overweight is defined as a BMI of 25–29.9 kg/m^2, and obesity is defined as a BMI $\geq$30 kg/m^2.[13]

Abdominal Obesity

Excess abdominal fat is an independent predictor of cardiovascular risk and morbidity.[13] Measuring waist circumference is one method used to identify high-risk individuals. Men with a waist circumference measuring more than 40 inches (>102 cm) and women measuring more than 35 inches (>88 cm) have an increased risk of obesity-associated complications.[13]

Physical Inactivity

It is estimated that 40% of the U.S. population is sedentary.[14] This lifestyle predisposes individuals to obesity, hypertension, hyperlipidemia, and diabetes.[14] Data from the Framingham Heart Study and other clinical trials have demonstrated that physical inactivity increases the risk of CHD.[15,16]

Psychosocial Factors

Various social factors have been associated with an increased risk of CHD.[14,17] These factors include social isolation, depression, hostility, low education level, and work-related stress. Individuals with a low education level may be less likely to modify their lifestyles to reduce cardiovascular risk. Work-related stress increases catecholamines, which can increase heart rate and blood pressure.

Ethnic Characteristics

The risk of CHD varies among different ethnic groups.[2] This may be due to differences in the physical and cultural environments as well as genetics. For example, differences may exist between ethnic groups in the types of food consumed, availability of food, or meal frequency. There may be differences in attitudes about ideal body image and the use of food in social settings. Genetics may also play a role as evidenced by the high rate of diabetes mellitus in Mexican and Native Americans and the high rate of hypertension in African-Americans.

Small, Dense LDL

LDL cholesterol has clearly been associated with an increased atherosclerotic risk; however, it is not the only factor that plays a role in the development of CHD. Multiple subclasses of LDL particles have been identified. The presence of small, dense LDL particles is associated with an increased risk of CHD and is often accompanied by elevated intermediate-density LDL cholesterol (IDL), low HDL cholesterol, elevated triglycerides, and insulin resistance.[18,19] Individuals with this "atherogenic lipoprotein profile" have a threefold increased risk of CHD and are at increased risk for the development of diabetes mellitus.[19] The presence of small, dense LDL particles cannot be detected by routine cholesterol screening and sophisticated laboratory testing methods must be used, which can be costly.

Lipoprotein(a)

Epidemiologic and clinic trials have demonstrated that elevated lipoprotein(a) LPa is associated with an increased risk for atherosclerotic disorders including coronary artery disease, peripheral vascular disease, and cerebrovascular disease.[19,20] LPa is larger and more dense than LDL cholesterol and binds more strongly than LDL to arterial walls. It is also taken up by macrophages more easily, leading to foam cell formation and oxidative damage.[20] LPa is structurally similar to plasminogen, which may be responsible for its pathogenic mechanisms.[20]

Fibrinogen

Fibrinogen is a prothrombotic factor and a major determinant of platelet aggregation and blood viscosity. Elevated fibrinogen levels have been associated with a higher incidence of CHD.[21] Some factors that can increase fibrinogen levels include cigarette smoking, diabetes mellitus, advancing age, inflammation, high dietary fat intake, oral contraceptives, menopause, and vascular damage.[21]

C-Reactive Protein

Local and systemic inflammation plays an important role in the initiation and progression of atherosclerosis. C-Reactive protein (CRP) is an acute phase reactant marker for underlying systemic inflammation and is found in atherosclerotic lesions. Elevated CRP levels have been found in patients with acute ischemia and are associated with increased cardiovascular risk.[22] A dose-response relationship exists between the level of CRP and the risk of CHD. Individuals are considered to be at low risk for cardiovascular disease when CRP levels are less than 1.0 mg/L, intermediate risk when CRP levels are between 1.0 and 3.0 mg/L, and high risk when CRP levels exceed 3.0 mg/L.[23] CRP can be measured during fasting or nonfasting states, and the measurement should be repeated once in stable patients.[23]

Homocysteine

Several prospective studies have noted an association between elevated plasma homocysteine levels and CHD risk.[24,25] The mechanism by which hyperhomocysteinemia contributes to vascular damage and cardiovascular disease is not completely understood. It also remains unclear what causes elevated homocysteine levels. Some theories include advancing age, systemic disease, vitamin deficiency, medications, and enzymatic deficiencies.[26]

Goals of Treatment

Studies have consistently shown a strong correlation between blood pressure and the risk of cardiovascular disease.[27] The primary goal when treating patients with hypertension is to reduce morbidity and mortality. This can be achieved by reducing blood pressure, controlling cardiovascular risk factors, and administering aspirin in appropriate patients.

Blood Pressure Control

It is important to establish a goal blood pressure for every patient. According to the seventh report of the Joint National Committee on Prevention, Detection, Evaluation, and Treatment of High Blood Pressure (JNC 7), the goal blood pressure for the majority of patients is less than 140/90 mm Hg.[4] For patients with diabetes and chronic kidney disease, the goal blood pressure is less than 130/80 mm Hg. Chronic kidney disease is defined by either (1) an estimated glomerular filtration rate (GFR) of less than 60 ml/min per 1.73 m^2, or (2) the presence of albuminuria (>300 mg/day).[4] It is often difficult for patients with isolated systolic hypertension to achieve these blood pressure goals. Therefore, a partial blood pressure reduction may be an acceptable interim goal.

Risk Factor Modification

In addition to establishing blood pressure goals, it is important to establish goals for individuals with concurrent cardiovascular risk factors. Cigarette smoking is one of the most important modifiable risk factors. Current smokers should be encouraged to quit at every visit, and pharmacologic therapies should be offered. Treatment of dyslipidemia and diabetes is critical, and **Tables 4-3 and 4-4** list the

Table 4-3.
LDL Cholesterol and Non-HDL Cholesterol Goals[6]

Risk Category	LDL, mg/dl	Non-HDL, mg/dl
CHD and CHD risk equivalents* (10-year risk for CHD >20%)	<100	<130
Multiple (2+) risk factors	<130	<160
0–1 risk factor	<160	<190

*CHD risk equivalents: peripheral arterial disease, abdominal aortic aneurysm, symptomatic carotid artery disease, diabetes, multiple risk factors conferring a 10-year risk for CHD >20%.

Table 4-4.
Goals for Type 2 Diabetes Mellitus*[10]

Biochemical Index	Goal
A1c	<7%
Preprandial plasma glucose	90–130 mg/dl
Peak postprandial plasma glucose	<180 mg/dl

*Goals should be individualized.

current goals of therapy for these disease states. All overweight and obese patients should be encouraged to lose weight. The goals of weight loss include prevention of further weight gain, reduction in body weight, and maintenance of lower body weight over the long term.[13]

The American Heart Association has published recommendations for health care providers on how to implement physical activity for primary and secondary prevention of CHD.[28] Small, dense LDL is not routinely monitored; however, sophisticated laboratory tests are available and may be beneficial in high-risk patients. Effective treatments for modifying small, dense LDL include lifestyle modifications, niacin, and fibrates.[19] There is a lack of data evaluating the effects of lowering fibrinogen levels on the risk of CHD. However, several therapies have been shown to decrease fibrinogen and include ticlopidine, β-blockers, and various lifestyle modifications (physical activity, smoking cessation, and limitation of dietary fat).[21]

Measurement of CRP may become a valuable tool in the future to identify individuals at high risk for CHD. Lifestyle modifications, HMG CoA reductase inhibitors, fibrates, nicotinic acid, and aspirin have been shown to lower CRP levels; however, there is a lack of clinical data to support a

reduction in cardiovascular morbidity and mortality.[23,29] The B vitamins (folic acid, B_{12}, and B_6) play a major role in homocysteine metabolism and clearance. Dietary consumption and supplementation with B vitamins have been shown to lower homocysteine levels.[25] However, it remains unclear if lowering homocysteine levels will reduce the risk of CHD.

Antiplatelet Therapy

As mentioned previously, the primary goal when treating patients with hypertension is to reduce morbidity and mortality. In addition to blood pressure control and risk factor modification, this can be achieved with the administration of aspirin. Secondary prevention trials have conclusively shown that aspirin reduces the risk of recurrent myocardial infarction, stroke, and cardiovascular death in patients with established CHD.[30] This benefit is independent of age, gender, and cardiovascular risk factors. Therefore, it is recommended that aspirin be administered in all patients with established CHD at a dose of 75–162.5 mg daily.[30] Several primary prevention trials have also demonstrated that aspirin significantly reduced the risk of a first myocardial infarction in healthy and high-risk patients without CHD.[31–33]

Based on the results of these studies, the Sixth ACCP Consensus Conference on Antithrombotic Therapy guidelines recommend administering aspirin in men and women over the age of 50 with at least one major risk factor for CHD (including hypertension).[30] Aspirin therapy is not recommended in individuals less than 50 years of age without a previous history of myocardial infarction, stroke, or transient ischemic attack.[30] The JNC 7 guidelines also recommend the use of low-dose aspirin (i.e., 81 mg per day) in patients with hypertension. However, its use should be limited to those patients whose blood pressure is controlled, due to the increased risk of hemorrhagic stroke in patients with uncontrolled hypertension.[4]

Patient Involvement When Establishing Treatment Goals

As mentioned in Chapter 1, hypertension can be a relatively asymptomatic disease. It is well known that treatments for hypertension are associated with many risks and adverse effects. They can also be very expensive for patients. When establishing treatment goals, it is important to share information with patients and actively involve them in the decision-making process. This approach will likely improve adherence and patient satisfaction.

The overall goal when treating hypertension is to reduce morbidity and mortality. This should be a common goal between patients and health care providers. Patients should be thoroughly educated on hypertension and the complications associated with the disease. If patients are unaware of the consequences of hypertension, they may be less likely to adhere to treatment recommendations. Patients should be informed that hypertension is a chronic medical condition that will require long-term changes in lifestyle and daily habits to maintain control. They should understand that pharmacologic therapy may need to be added, and this can be associated with adverse effects and increased costs.

In addition to discussing the sequelae of hypertension, patients should be informed about the contribution of other cardiovascular risk factors to overall CHD risk. The importance of modification of these factors should also be stressed. It is likely that many patients will have questions regarding their new diagnosis and should be given the opportunity to ask questions and voice their concerns.

It may take a significant amount of time for patients to meet their treatment goals. Interim goals can be established that may give patients a sense of accomplishment. Examples include interim blood pressure goals (particularly with isolated systolic hypertension in the elderly), 10% interim weight loss goal, and ongoing encouragement for smoking cessation despite recent failed attempts. Patients should also receive positive reinforcement on their progress toward their goals.

Key Points for Patients

- Patients have different blood pressure goals based on the presence of cardiovascular risk factors, target organ damage, and clinical cardiovascular disease.
- To reduce the risk of morbidity and mortality, blood pressure goals must be met and cardiovascular risk factors must be modified.
- Adequate education should be provided to patients about the consequences of hypertension and the importance of treatment.
- Patients should become involved in the decision-making process when treating hypertension and cardiovascular risk factors.

Patient Case

1 JR is a 67-year-old male who was recently diagnosed with hypertension. His past medical history is also significant for type 2 diabetes mellitus and tobacco abuse (one pack per day). He leads a relatively sedentary lifestyle. His current medications include metformin 500 mg BID and aspirin 81 mg QD. He weighs 120 kg and is 1.83 meters tall. His resting blood pressure and heart rate are 152/98 mm Hg and 72 BPM, respectively. His fasting labs taken this morning are as follows:

Total cholesterol = 199 mg/dl

HDL cholesterol = 32 mg/dl

Calculated LDL cholesterol = 146 mg/dl

Triglycerides = 102 mg/dl

A1c = 7.9 %

From your initial evaluation, how many risk factors does JR have for CHD?

JR has a total of eight risk factors for CHD, including hypertension, diabetes, and tobacco abuse. All are major risk factors for CHD. Other risk factors include his age (67 years old) and physical inactivity. Based on the laboratory information provided, his HDL cholesterol is low at 32 mg/dl and his LDL cholesterol is high at 146 mg/dl. His BMI is calculated at 35.8 kg/m² based on his height and weight.

What are the goals of therapy for JR?

- *Blood pressure <130/80 mm Hg*
- *LDL cholesterol <100 mg/dl*
- *A1c <7%*
- *Smoking cessation*
- *Physical activity*
- *Weight loss*

References

1. Cupples LA, D'Agostino RB. Some risk factors related to the annual incidence of cardiovascular disease and death using pooled repeated biennial measurements. Framingham heart study: 30-year follow-up. Washington, DC: U.S. Department of Health and Human Services, Public Health Service, National Heart, Lung, and Blood Institute, 1987; NIH document 87-2703.

2. Grundy SM, Pasternak R, Greenland P et al. Assessment of cardiovascular risk by use of multiple-risk-factor assessment equations. *Circulation.* 1999; 100:1481–92.

3. Smith SC, Greenland P, Grundy SM. Beyond secondary prevention: identifying the high-risk patient for primary prevention: executive summary. *Circulation.* 2000; 101:111–6.

4. The seventh report of the Joint National Committee on Prevention, Detection, Evaluation, and Treatment of High Blood Pressure. The JNC 7 report. *JAMA.* 2003; 289:2560–72.

5. 2003 European Society of Hypertension–European Society of Cardiology guidelines for the management of arterial hypertension. *J Hypertens.* 2003; 21:1011–53.

6. Expert Panel on Detection, Evaluation, and Treatment of High Blood Cholesterol in Adults. Executive summary of the third report of the National Cholesterol Education Program (NCEP) Expert Panel on Detection, Evaluation, and Treatment of High Blood Cholesterol in Adults (Adult Treatment Panel III). *JAMA.* 2001; 285:2486–97.

7. Jonas MA, Oates JA, Ockene JK et al. Statement on smoking and cardiovascular disease for health care professionals. American Heart Association. *Circulation.* 1992; 86:1664–9.

8. Taylor BV, Oudit GY, Kalman PG et at. Clinical and pathophysiological effects of active and passive smoking on the cardiovascular system. *Can J Cardiol.* 1998; 14:1129–39.

9. Austin MA, Hokanson JE, Edwards KL. Hypertriglyceridemia as a cardiovascular risk factor. *Am J Cardiol.* 1998; 81:7B–12B.

10. The Expert Committee on the Diagnosis and Classification of Diabetes Mellitus. American Diabetes Association: clinical practice recommendations 2003. *Diabetes Care.* 2003; 26:S1–156.

11. Haffner SM, Lehto S, Ronneman T et al. Mortality from coronary heart disease in subjects with type 2 diabetes and in nondiabetic subjects with and without prior myocardial infarction. *N Engl J Med.* 1998; 339:229–34.

12. Myers RH, Kiely DK, Cupples LA et al. Parental history is an independent risk factor for coronary artery disease: the Framingham study. *Am Heart J.* 1990; 120:963–9.

13. NHLBI Obesity Education Initiative. Clinical guidelines on the identification, evaluation, and treatment of overweight and obesity in adults. National Institutes of Health, National Heart, Lung, and Blood Institute. September 1998, NIH Publication no. 98-4083.

14. Robinson JF, Leon AS. The prevention of cardiovascular disease. Emphasis on secondary prevention. *Med Clin North Am.* 1994; 78:69–97.

15. U.S. Department of Health and Human Services. Physical activity and health: a report of the Surgeon General. Atlanta, GA: Department of Health and Human Services, Centers for Disease Control and Prevention, National Center for Chronic Disease Prevention and Health Promotion; 1996.

16. Kannel WB, Wilson PF, Blair SN. Epidemiological assessment of the role of physical activity and fitness in development of cardiovascular disease. *Am Heart J.* 1985; 109:876–85.

17. King KB. Psychologic and social aspects of cardiovascular disease. *Ann Behav Med.* 1997; 19:264–70.

18. Austin MA, Hokanson JE. Epidemiology of triglycerides, small dense low-density lipoprotein, and lipoprotein(a) as risk factors for coronary heart disease. *Med Clin North Am.* 1994; 78:99–115.

19. Superko HR. Did grandma give you heart disease? The new battle against coronary artery disease. *Am J Cardiol.* 1998; 82:34Q–46Q.

20. Dahlen GH, Stenlund H. Lp(a) lipoprotein is a major risk factor for cardiovascular disease: pathogenic mechanisms and clinical significance. *Clin Genet.* 1997; 52:272–80.

21. Maresca G, Di Blasio A, Marchioli R et al. Measuring plasma fibrinogen to predict stroke and myocardial infarction. *Arterioscler Thromb Vasc Biol.* 1999; 19:1368–77.

22. Patel VB, Robbins MA, Topol EJ. C-Reactive protein: a 'golden marker' for inflammation and coronary artery disease. *Cleve Clin J Med.* 2001; 68:535–7.

23. Ridker PM. Clinical application of C-reactive protein for cardiovascular disease detection and prevention. *Circulation.* 2003; 107:363–9.

24. Stampfer MJ, Malinow MR, Willett WC. A prospective study of plasma homocysteine and risk of myocardial infarction in US physicians. *JAMA.* 1992; 268:877–81.

25. Ottar N, Nordehaug JE, Refsum H. Plasma homocysteine levels and mortality in patients with coronary artery disease. *N Engl J Med.* 1997; 337:230–6.

26. Chai AU, Abrams J. Homocysteine: A new cardiac risk factor? *Clin Cardiol.* 2001; 24:80–4.

27. Kannel WB. Blood pressure as a cardiovascular risk factor. *JAMA.* 1996; 275:1571–6.

28. Statement on exercise: benefits and recommendations for physical activity programs for all Americans. A statement for health professionals by the Committee on Exercise and Cardiac Rehabilitation of the Council on Clinical Cardiology, American Heart Association. American Heart Association. *Circulation.* 1996; 94:857–62.

29. Kreisberg R, Oberman A. Medical management of hyperlipidemia/dyslipidemia. *J Clin Endocrinol Metab.* 2003; 88:2445–61.

30. Cairns JA, Therous P, Lewis D et al. Antithrombotic agents in coronary artery disease. *Chest.* 2001; 119:228S–52S.

31. Steering Committee of the Physicians' Health Study Research Group. Final report on the aspirin component of the ongoing Physicians' Health Study. *N Engl J Med.* 1989; 321:129–35.

32. Peto R, Gray R, Collins R et al. Randomized trial of prophylactic daily aspirin in British male doctors. *BMJ.* 1988; 926:313–6.

33. Hansson L, Zanchetti A, Carruthers SG et al. Effects of intensive blood-pressure lowering and low-dose aspirin in patients with hypertension: principal results of the Hypertension Optimal Treatment (HOT) randomized trial. *Lancet.* 1998; 351:1755–62.

Chapter 5:

Pharmacology of Antihypertensive Agents

Alan H. Mutnick

Clinical Highlights

- What are the most recent drug treatment recommendations for hypertension?
- What are the primary mechanisms of action for the major antihypertensive classes of drugs?
- What are the primary adverse drug reactions associated with the use of the major antihypertensive classes?

After establishing treatment goals for patients with hypertension based on risk stratification, it is necessary to select the most cost-effective antihypertensive regimen in order to reduce blood pressure with minimal adverse effects. In most situations, professional experience will play a major role in the evaluation of treatment options. However, consensus guidelines have been developed that allow the clinician to integrate professional experience with established guidelines developed through appropriate reviews of evidence-based treatment modalities.

Antihypertensive therapy involves pharmacologic as well as nonpharmacologic treatments. **Table 5-1** provides a list of currently available agents for each class of antihypertensive drugs.[1-3] An important role for pharmacists to assume in the treatment of hypertension is to have a keen appreciation for the similarities and differences that exist among the available pharmacologic treatments. The pharmacist's ability to relate mechanisms of action and side effect profiles of drugs to individual clinical needs and goals for each specific patient is a vital role that needs to be carried out for the other members of the health care team.

It has been estimated that 50–70% of antihypertensive treatment regimens are changed and/or discontinued within the first 6 months.[4] These high percentages are believed to be due to a combination of adverse drug effects, cost of drugs, inadequate control, changes in clinician, dissatisfaction with other aspects of care, and an overall lack of understanding of the risks of target organ damage.[4] Consequently, a fundamental knowledge by the pharmacist of the manner in which antihypertensives work and the primary side effects which

they possess would be expected to improve compliance with treatment regimens. **Table 5-2** provides a comparison of the actions, adverse drug reactions, drug interactions, and recommended dosing guidelines for currently available antihypertensives.[2,3,5-9]

Angiotensin-Converting Enzyme Inhibitors

The angiotensin-converting enzyme (ACE, kininase II) works by cleaving off the terminal dipeptide from angiotensin I with the resultant production of angiotensin II, which is a potent vasoconstrictor acting directly on vascular smooth muscle cells.[10] Angiotensin II possesses additional stimulatory effects on aldosterone and antidiuretic hormone, resulting in fluid volume expansion (sodium retention) as well as fluid retention.[10]

ACE inhibitors decrease systemic vascular resistance but have little effect on heart rate.[10] This benefit is in contrast to other vasodilators such as the calcium channel blockers and direct-acting vasodilators and might represent an effect which ACE inhibitors have on barreceptors as well as on the sympathetic nervous system. In normotensive and hypertensive subjects with normal left ventricular function, they have little effect on cardiac output and pulmonary capillary wedge pressure. ACE inhibitors effectively lower the mean, systolic, and diastolic pressures in hypertensive patients as well as in salt-depleted and volume-depleted normotensive subjects.[10] The change in blood pressure correlates with pretreatment plasma renin activity

Table 5-1.
Currently Available Antihypertensives[1-3]

Antihypertensive Class	Available Agents: Generic/Tradename
Thiazide diuretics	Bendroflumethiazide/Naturetin® Chlorothiazide/Diuril® Chlorthalidone/Hygroton® Hydrochlorothiazide/ HydroDIURIL® Hydroflumethiazide/Saluron® Indapamide/Lozol® Methyclothiazide/Enduron® Metolazone/Zaroxolyn®, Mykrox® Polythiazide/Renese® Trichlormethiazide/Naqua®
Loop diuretics	Bumetanide/Bumex® Ethacrynic acid/Edecrin® Furosemide/Lasix® Torsemide/Demadex®
Potassium-sparing diuretics	Amiloride/Midamor® Spironolactone/Aldactone® Triamterene/Dyrenium®
Vasodilators (direct acting)	Diazoxide/Hyperstat®, Proglycem® Hydralazine HCl/Apresoline® Minoxidil/Loniten® Sodium nitroprusside/ Nitropress®
ACE inhibitors	Benazepril HCl/Lotensin® Captopril/Capoten® Enalaprilat/Vasotec® I.V. Enalapril maleate/Vasotec® Fosinopril sodium/Monopril® Lisinopril/Prinivil®, Zestril® Moexipril/Univasc® Perindopril erbumine/Aceon® Quinapril HCl/Accupril® Ramipril/Altace® Trandolapril/Mavik®
ARBs	Candesartan cilexetil/Atacand® Eprosartan mesylate/Teveten® Irbesartan/Avapro® Losartan potassium/Cozaar® Olmesartan medoxomil/ Benicar® Telmisartan/Micardis® Valsartan/Diovan®
Sympatholytics *β-Adrenergic blocking agents*	Acebutolol HCl/Sectral® Atenolol/Tenormin® Betaxolol HCl/Kerlone® Bisoprolol/Zebeta® Carteolol/Cartrol® Carvedilol/Coreg® Labetalol HCl/Normodyne®, Trandate®

(continued)

Table 5-1. *(continued)*
Currently Available Antihypertensives[1-3]

Antihypertensive Class	Available Agents: Generic/Tradename
Sympatholytics *β-Adrenergic blocking agents (cont'd)*	Metoprolol/Lopressor® (tartrate), Toprol® (succinate) Nadolol/Corgard® Penbutolol/Levatol® Pindolol/Visken® Propranolol HCl/Inderal®, various Timolol maleate/Blocadren®
Centrally acting α-agonists	Clonidine/Catapres® Guanabenz/Wytensin® Guanfacine/Tenex® Methyldopa/Aldomet®
Postganglionic adrenergic neuron blockers	Reserpine/various
α-Adrenergic blocking agents	Doxazosin mesylate/Cardura® Prazosin HCl/Minipress® Terazosin HCl/Hytrin®
CCBs	**Benzothiazepine derivatives** Diltiazem/Cardizem®, Dilacor®, Tiazac®, various **Diphenylalkylamine derivatives** Verapamil/Calan®, Isoptin®, various **Dihydropyridines** Amlodipine/Norvasc® Felodipine/Plendil® Isradipine/DynaCirc® Nicardipine/Cardene® Nifedipine/ Adalat ® CC, Procardia XL® Nisoldipine/Sular®

along with angiotensin levels. Consequently, the greatest reduction in blood pressure occurs in those patients with the highest plasma renin activity.[10]

One area that has generated controversy is the use of ACE inhibitors in patients with renal insufficiency.[11,12] ACE inhibitors are not nephrotoxic, and baseline serum creatinine levels of up to 3.0 mg/dl are generally considered safe.[12] The manufacturers provide recommendations for initiating treatment by suggesting dosage titration upward in a slow fashion. An increase in serum creatinine of 20% is not uncommon and is not a cause for discontinuing the medication. For any higher increase, consideration should be given to contacting a nephrologist for follow-up. Additionally, during the first

Table 5-2.
Comparison of Anti-Hypertensive Agents[2,3,5-9]

Diuretics

Therapeutic Class	Mechanism of Action	Common ADRs	Drug Interactions	Special Considerations	Dosing Guidelines
Thiazides	Increase urinary excretion of sodium and water by inhibiting sodium and chloride reabsorption in the distal convoluted (renal) tubules. Increase urinary excretion of potassium and, to a lesser extent, bicarbonate. Decreased peripheral vascular resistance.	Fatigue, headache, palpitations, vertigo, and transitory impotence. Postural hypotension, alterations in fluid and electrolytes (e.g., hypokalemia, hypomagnesemia, hypercalcemia, hyperglycemia).	NSAIDs diminish the antihypertensive effects of the thiazide diuretics. Long-term use may reduce lithium excretion. Calcium-containing antacids may cause hypercalcemia.	Fluid losses must be evaluated and monitored to prevent dehydration, uric acid retention may occur; this is potentially significant in patients who are predisposed to gout and related disorders. Blood glucose levels may increase, which may be significant in the patient with diabetes. Calcium levels may increase because of the potential for retaining calcium ions. Patients with known allergies to sulfa-type drugs should be questioned to determine the significance of the allergy.	Bendroflumethiazide 2.5–15.0 mg daily Benzthiazide 50–150 mg daily Chlorothiazide 500–2000 mg daily Chlorthalidone 15–200 mg daily Hydrochlorothiazide 12.5–50 mg daily Hydroflumethiazid 25–100 mg daily Indapamide 1.25–5.0 mg daily Methyclothiazide 2.5–10.0 mg daily Metolazone 5–20.0 mg daily Polythiazide 1–4 mg daily Quinethazone 50–200 mg daily Trichlormethiazide 2–4 mg daily
Loop diuretics	Act primarily in the ascending loop of Henle to decrease sodium reabsorption. Their action is more intense but of shorter duration (1–4 hours) than that of the thiazides.	Dehydration, hypotension, hypokalemia, hyperglycemia as with thiazides. Transient deafness.	NSAIDs may decrease diuretic effect. Cholestyramine decreases furosemide absorption.	Renal function must be monitored closely for signs of hypovolemia. BUN and serum creatinine levels should be checked routinely.	Bumetanide 0.5–10.0 mg daily Ethacrynic acid 50–200 mg daily Furosemide 80–600 mg daily Torsemide 5.0–10 mg daily

(continued)

Table 5-2. (continued)
Comparison of Anti-Hypertensive Agents[2,3,5-9]

Therapeutic Class	Mechanism of Action	Common ADRs	Drug Interactions	Special Considerations	Dosing Guidelines
Diuretics					
Potassium-sparing diuretics	Act in the distal convoluted tubule of the kidney by promoting excretion of sodium and water with a resultant retention in potassium.	Hyperkalemia, dehydration, hyponatremia. Estrogen-like side effects (spironolactone) such as gynecomastia, decreased libido. Nausea, vomiting, diarrhea dizziness (triamterene).	Coadministration with ACE inhibitors or potassium supplements significantly increases the risk of hyperkalemia. Spironolactone increases digoxin levels. Indomethacin and other NSAIDs may decrease renal function when combine with triamterene.	Avoid in patients with acute renal failure, use with caution in patients with impaired renal function because they can retain potassium. Triamterene should not be used in patients with a history of kidney stones or hepatic disease. Hyperkalemia is a major risk, requiring routine monitoring of serum electrolytes. BUN and serum creatinine levels should be checked routinely to signal excess potassium retention and impaired renal function.	Amiloride 5–10 mg daily Spironolactone 25–100 mg daily Triamterene 100–300 mg daily Eplerenone 50–100 mg daily
Direct-acting vasodilators	Act by directly relaxing peripheral vascular smooth muscle—arterial, venous, or both.	Hydralazine: Reflex tachycardia, angina. Drug-induced systemic lupus erythematosus. Fatigue, malaise, low-grade fever, and joint aches may signal SLE. Other adverse effects may include headache, peripheral neuropathy, nausea, vomiting, fluid retention, and postural hypotension. Minoxidil: increase in heart rate, cardiac output, and renin secretion. Sodium and water retention. Hypertrichosis, i.e., excessive hair growth.	NSAIDs may decrease hypotensive effect of hydralazine.	The direct vasodilators should not be used alone owing to increases in plasma renin activity, cardiac output, and heart rate. Hydralazine: Fatigue, malaise, low-grade fever, and joint aches may signal SLE. Minoxidil: patients should be monitored for fluid accumulation and signs of cardiac decompensation.	Hydralazine 50–300 mg in 2 doses. Minoxidil 5–100 mg in 1 or 2 doses.

(continued)

Table 5-2. *(continued)*
Comparison of Anti-Hypertensive Agents[2,3,5–9]

Therapeutic Class	Mechanism of Action	Common ADRs	Drug Interactions	Special Considerations	Dosing Guidelines
Centrally acting α-agonists	Stimulation of α_2 receptor causes decrease sympathetic outflow to the kidneys, heart, and peripheral vasculature, and a resultant decrease in peripheral vascular resistance, systolic and diastolic blood pressure, and heart rate.	Drowsiness, sedation, dry mouth, fatigue, orthostatic hypotension, and dizziness.	Heterocyclic antidepressants may decrease hypotensive effect of clonidine; clonidine may inhibit antiparkinson effect of levodopa; prazosin may decrease effect of clonidine; verapamil may cause additive hypotension and conduction disturbances. Methyldopa may potentiate tolbutamide and lithium; may increase confusion with haloperidol use; levodopa and methyldopa together enhance each other's effects.	Hypotension and dizziness most prominent during initial days of therapy and with dosing adjustments, particularly in the elderly. Caution in these patients when starting therapy or adjusting doses.	Clonidine Average daily dose is 0.2–2.4 mg in 2 doses. Methyldopa Average daily dose is 500 mg–2.0 g in 2–4 doses. Guanabenz Average daily doses is 4–64 mg in 2 doses. Guanfacine 1–3 mg in 1 dose.
β-adrenergic blockers	Block the agonistic effects of sympathetic neurotransmitters through a competitive mechanism on receptor binding sites. Additional properties for select agents include Relatively Cardioselective, Intrinsic Sympathomimetic Activity.	Hypotension, CHF, light-headedness, cold extremities bradycardia, fatigue bronchospasm, peripheral artery insufficiency, decrease in exercise tolerance, depression.	β-blockers may prolong hypoglycemic episodes and inhibit tachycardia; β-blockers have additive effects with diltiazem/verapamil on reduced electrical conduction and reduced cardiac contractility; cimetidine may increase effects of propranolol; combination with clonidine may result in hypertensive reactions. NSAIDs may reduce hypotensive effect.	Patients must be monitored for signs and symptoms of cardiac decompensation, ECGs should be monitored for conduction abnormalities. Relative cardioselectivity is dose-dependent and is lost as dosages are increased. No agent is completely safe in patients with bronchospastic disease. Suddenly stopping β-blocker therapy puts the patient at risk i.e., exacerbated anginal attacks, particularly in patients with coronary artery disease. Diabetes β-blockers can mask hypoglycemic symptoms, such as tachycardia.	See Table 5-4

(continued)

Table 5-2. (continued)
Comparison of Anti-Hypertensive Agents[2,3,5-9]

Therapeutic Class	Mechanism of Action	Common ADRs	Drug Interactions	Special Considerations	Dosing Guidelines
β-adrenergic blockers				Raynaud's phenomenon or peripheral vascular disease. Vasoconstriction can occur. Impotence and decreased libido may result in reduced patient adherence.	See Table 5-3
Angiotensin-Converting Enzyme Inhibitors (ACEIs)	Inhibition of angiotensin-converting enzyme resulting in reduced angiotensin II levels and aldosterone secretion.	Dry, hacking cough, skin rash, dizziness, angioedema, hyperkalemia.	ACEIs may increase lithium levels; NSAIDs may reduce the anti-hypertensive effect of ACEIs. Potassium supplements—may exacerbate ACEI induced hyperkalemia.	Avoid in patients with bilateral renal artery stenosis. Avoid in pregnancy. Discontinue if angioedema develops. Monitor initiation of therapy closely in patients with renal insufficiency.	
Angiotensin-II receptor antagonists (ARBs)	High affinity to the angiotensin-type$_1$ (AT$_1$) receptors resulting in reduced blood pressure by inhibiting the actions of angiotensin II. Unlike ACEIs, which increase bradykinin levels through their inhibitory effect on the converting enzyme (kininase II), ARBs believed to have less side effects as compared to ACEIs.	Headache, dizziness, nasal congestion, cough, and fatigue. Hyperkalemia, neutropenia, angioedema, rash, reversible renal dysfunction.	Potassium supplements—may exacerbate ACEI induced hyperkalemia.	Avoid in patients with bilateral renal artery stenosis. Avoid in pregnancy. Discontinue if angioedema develops. Monitor initiation of therapy closely in patients with renal insufficiency.	Candesartan 8–32 mg in 1–2 doses Eprosartan 600–800 mg in 1 dose Irbesartan 150–300 mg in 1 dose Losartan 25–100 mg in 1–2 doses Olmesartan 20–40 mg in 1 dose Telmisartan 20–80 mg in 1 dose Valsartan 80–320 mg in 1 dose
Postganglionic adrenergic neuron blockers (Reserpine)	Works at the postganglionic neurons by depleting catecholamines resulting in reduced sympathetic actions and a decrease in cardiac output and peripheral vascular resistance.	Dizziness, lethargy, nasal congestion, GI disturbance (ulcer, abdominal pain, diarrhea), nightmares, and mental depression (particularly in elderly with potential for suicidal behavior).		A history of depression is a contraindication for reserpine. Drug-induced depression may linger for months after the last dose. Peptic ulcer is also a contraindication for using reserpine.	Reserpine Average dose is 0.05–0.25 mg in 1 dose

(continued)

51

Table 5-2. (continued)
Comparison of Anti-Hypertensive Agents[2,3,5–9]

Therapeutic Class	Mechanism of Action	Common ADRs	Drug Interactions	Special Considerations	Dosing Guidelines
α-Adrenergic blocking agents (doxazosin, prazosin, and terazosin)	Blocking peripheral postsynaptic α₁-receptor, resulting in peripheral vasodilation and a reduction in peripheral vascular resistance without a reduction in cardiac output.	First-dose orthostatic hypotensive, dizziness, lightheadedness, syncope, weakness, palpitations, and headache.	NSAIDs may reduce hypotensive effects of prazosin. β-blockers and verapamil may increase postural effects of prazosin. α-adrenergic blocking agents may decrease the hypotensive effects of clonidine.	In the ALLHAT Trial, doxazosin was shown to increase the risk (25% incidence) for congestive heart failure, stroke, and coronary heart disease in predisposed patients.	Prazosin 2–30 mg in 2 doses Terazosin 1–20 mg in 1 dose Doxazosin 1–16 mg in 1 dose
Calcium channel blockers (CCBs)	Peripheral vasodilation and a resultant decrease in peripheral vascular resistance.	Headache, dizziness, peripheral edema, tachycardia (nifedipine and other diltiazem: 120–360 mg in two doses dihydropyridines), gingival hyperplasia, constipation, AV block, bradycardia, and signs of cardiac decompensation (non-dihydropyridine derivatives).	β-blockers plus CCBs may have an additive effect on inducing CHF and bradycardia. AV nodal conduction may be depressed when patients are given β-blockers with verapamil and diltiazem.	Diltiazem and verapamil must be used with extreme caution if at all in patients with conductive disturbances involving the SA or AV node. Rapid acting nifedipine use has been associated with flushing, headache, and peripheral edema, and increased risk of ischemic events, and the current recommendation is to avoid its use if at all possible. Verapamil has been associated with a significant degree of constipation, which must be treated to prevent stool straining and nonadherence.	See Table 5-5

4 weeks of treatment, serum potassium and creatinine levels should be monitored closely.[12]

ACE inhibitor therapy has been associated with a syndrome of *"functional renal insufficiency,"* which most commonly develops shortly after initiation of therapy but has been observed after months or years of therapy.[11] This form of acute renal failure is not attributed to the effects of ACE inhibitors on the kidneys directly, but it is most likely to occur when renal perfusion pressure cannot be sustained due to significant decreases in mean arterial pressure.[11] As long as renal perfusion pressure is sufficient and volume depletion is not severe, ACE inhibitors have been shown to improve renal hemodynamics with a resultant improvement in renal salt excretion. Unfortunately, angiotensin II is necessary for maintenance of glomerular filtration rates during states of significant volume depletion, and the ACE inhibitors by reducing angiotensin II levels are able to cause a decrease in glomerular filtration rates with a resultant onset of oliguric or anuric renal failure.[11]

Conditions causing renal hypoperfusion such as systemic hypotension, high-grade renal artery stenosis, extracellular fluid volume contraction (dehydration), administration of vasoconstrictor agents (e.g., nonsteroidal anti-inflammatory drugs or cyclosporine), and congestive heart failure have been shown to represent risk factors for the development of functional renal insufficiency in patients receiving ACE inhibitors.[11] These conditions typically increase renin secretion or angiotensin II production. When these conditions occur in patients receiving ACE inhibitors, angiotensin II formation and its effects on renal dynamics are diminished, and the glomerular filtration rate may decrease.

Adequate monitoring of patients who are prone to functional renal insufficiency can identify patients early enough to avoid withholding ACE inhibitor therapy due to concerns of the potential for renal impairment.[11] Monitoring of patients would include fluid status, baseline blood pressure readings, and follow-up serum creatinine and potassium levels.[11] Additionally, the discontinuation of diuretic therapy prior to initiation of ACE inhibitors will reduce concerns for the development of dehydration.

Though controversial, ACE inhibitors are not contraindicated in patients with renal impairment, but their use requires a thorough understanding of the pathophysiological mechanisms and common risk factors for ACE inhibitor-induced renal insufficiency.[11] This will ensure the use of preventive strategies that will reduce the likelihood of the development of renal insufficiency and will permit the use of these agents, although perhaps in a more restricted manner. **Table 5-3** provides a comparison of recommended dosing for the ACE inhibitors currently available.[2,3,13]

Angiotensin II Receptor Antagonists

Four different types of angiotensin II receptors (ARBs) have been identified throughout the human body (AT_1, AT_2, AT_3, and AT_4).[14] AT_1 receptor effects include, but are not limited to, vasoconstriction, increased sodium retention, suppression of renin secretion, increased vasopressin release, and activation of sympathetic activity.

Several ARBs are available for clinical use in the treatment of hypertension, and all work through their high affinity to the AT_1 receptors with little affinity for AT_2 receptors. Consequently, the ARBs reduce blood pressure by inhibiting the actions of angiotensin II, similar to the ACE inhibitors. The ARBs have a more specific blockade of the renin-

Table 5-3.

Comparison of Currently Available Oral ACE Inhibitors in the Treatment of Hypertension[2,3,13]

Drug	Usual Dose Range* Total mg/day (Frequency per Day)	Maximum Effective Dose
Benazepril HCl	10–40 mg daily (1 or 2)	80 mg daily
Captopril	25–100 mg daily (2 or 3)	450 mg daily
Enalapril	2.5–40 mg daily (1 or 2)	40 mg daily
Fosinopril sodium	10–40 mg daily (1)	80 mg daily
Lisinopril	10–40 mg daily (1)	80 mg daily
Moexipril HCl	7.5–30 mg daily (1)	30 mg daily
Perindopril erbumine	4–8 mg daily (1 or 2)	16 mg daily
Quinapril HCl	10–40 mg daily (1)	80 mg daily
Ramipril	2.5–20 mg daily (1)	20 mg daily
Trandolapril	1–4 mg daily (1)	8 mg daily

*The doses listed represent the normal maintenance dose range. Initiation of therapy usually begins with doses in the lower usual dose range, and lower than normal doses are recommended for those patients currently receiving a diuretic.

angiotensin system and have been shown to have better tolerability when compared to ACE inhibitors.[14] Unlike the ACE inhibitors, which increase bradykinin levels through their inhibitory effect on the converting enzyme (kininase II) believed to play an important role in various side effects associated with ACE inhibitors, the ARBs appear to have a side effect profile similar to that of placebo. ARBs do not produce a cough and might represent an alternative treatment option in a patient maintained adequately on an ACE inhibitor but presenting with cough.

The ARBs have been evaluated in the treatment of mild-to-moderate hypertension and have been shown to be as effective as ACE inhibitors, calcium channel blockers, β-adrenergic blockers, and diuretics in the treatment of mild-to-moderate hypertension.[14] The ARBs (candesartan, eprosartan, irbesartan, losartan, olmesartan, telmisartan, and valsartan) share the same mechanism of action.[14] However, they do possess differing pharmacokinetic profiles which accounts for differences in efficacy, likely due to differences among duration of action as well as specific doses used clinically.[14] Side effects associated with the use of ARBs include fatigue, gastrointestinal disturbances, hyperkalemia, hypotension in patients who are volume depleted, and the slight possibility of angioedema of the face, tongue, and glottis.

Studies documenting the value of ARBs on morbidity and mortality in the hypertensive population are necessary to provide data comparable to the ACE inhibitors as well as diuretics and α-adrenergic blockers.

α-Adrenergic Blocking Agents

The pharmacologic effects of doxazosin, prazosin, and terazosin are believed to be due to the blocking action of the agents on the peripheral postsynaptic α_1-receptor. This effect results in peripheral vasodilation and a resultant decrease in peripheral vascular resistance without a reduction in cardiac output. Unlike other peripheral vasodilators (i.e., hydralazine), which result in reflex tachycardia, balanced arteriole/venous dilation does not appear to result in the same degree of reflex tachycardia.[1]

A *first-dose orthostatic hypotensive reaction* has been described for these agents and is believed to be dose dependent; the use of small doses upon

initiating therapy reduces its occurrence. Other side effects include dizziness, lightheadedness, syncope, weakness, palpitations, and headache. Patients predisposed to orthostatic hypotension include those who are volume depleted, those on sodium-restricted diets, and the elderly.[1]

The Antihypertensive and Lipid-Lowering Treatment to Prevent Heart Attack Trial (ALLHAT) randomly allocated patients to receive either the diuretic chlorthalidone in one of two doses or doxazosin in one of two doses.[15] The doxazosin arm of the trial was discontinued early because doxazosin recipients had a higher risk for stroke and combined cardiovascular disease as compared to those patients in the chlorthalidone study arm. Cardiovascular disease included angina, congestive heart failure, coronary revascularization, and peripheral artery disease, and the rate of congestive heart failure (CHF) alone was doubled in the doxazosin group as compared to the chlorthalidone group.[15] Therefore, the role for α-adrenergic blocking agents appears to be limited to those patients with benign prostatic hypertrophy.

β-Adrenergic Blockers

β-Adrenergic blocking agents work by blocking the agonistic effects of sympathetic neurotransmitters through a competitive mechanism on receptor binding sites.[1] Though the predominant mechanism of action for all β-adrenergic blockers is at the β-receptor site, additional pharmacologic effects have been described for several agents in the class, including *relatively cardioselective properties* and *intrinsic sympathomimetic activity*.

Relatively cardioselective refers to those agents having their predominant effect on the β_1-receptor within cardiac tissue resulting in reduced heart rate and little effect on other β-receptors. An example would be the β_2-receptors located in the lung which when blocked result in bronchoconstriction. *Relative* refers to the preference for such agents to occupy the β_1-receptor, as compared to propranolol, but as doses of these agents are increased, there is the tendency to block β_2-receptors as well. Metoprolol, atenolol, acebutolol, betaxolol, bisoprolol, and esmolol have been described as relatively cardioselective β-adrenergic blockers.

Intrinsic sympathomimetic activity (ISA) or partial agonist activity refers to those agents that are able to stimulate β_1-receptors under the appropriate circumstances while at the same time blocking the effects of endogenous catecholamines, in order to prevent a pure β-response in various organ systems. An agent with ISA activity might have the ability to prevent a patient from becoming significantly bradycardic, due to the weak stimulation of β_1-receptors when the heart rate decreases to a low; an agent with ISA activity might have the ability to prevent an *acute bronchospastic* effect through the stimulation of β_2-receptors in the lung, which would prevent such spasm. Pindolol, carteolol, penbutalol, and acebutolol have been described as possessing ISA.

In the treatment of hypertension, possible mechanisms of action for the β-receptor blockers include the ability to reduce cardiac output, decrease sympathetic impulses to the peripheral vasculature, and inhibit renin release from the juxta-glomerular apparatus within the kidney.[1] **Table 5-4** lists the β-adrenergic blockers currently available and compares them based on recommended doses, pharmacologic effects, and route of elimination.[2,3,6,7]

Calcium Channel Blockers

The calcium channel blockers (CCBs) are considered alternative drugs for the initial treatment of hypertension in select patient populations unable to take diuretics or β-adrenergic receptor blockers, such as patients with angina who also have bronchospastic disease or Raynaud's disease. Currently, the agents are available for the treatment of hypertension and are divided into three different chemical groups: benzothiazepine derivatives (diltiazem), diphenylalkylamine derivatives (verapamil), and dihydropyridine derivatives (amlodipine, felodipine, isradipine, nicardipine, nifedipine, and nisoldipine). **Table 5-5** provides the currently available CCBs and compares them based on suggested doses, routes of elimination, and relevant drug–food interactions.[2,3,5,8,9] Another CCB, bepridil, is not currently indicated in the treatment of hypertension and is primarily used in the treatment of angina pectoris.

The CCBs lower blood pressure by causing peripheral vasodilation and a resultant decrease in peripheral vascular resistance.[1] However, the three chemical groups have different hemodynamic effects. Dihydropyridine derivatives have a more selective effect on vascular smooth muscle as compared to effects on the myocardium and act primarily as vasodilators; they are associated with reflex tachycardia, similar to other peripheral vasodilators (i.e., hydralazine). The diphenylalkylamine derivative verapamil is less selective for peripheral smooth muscle, but it has a more direct effect on the myocardium to depress electrical conduction through the sinoatrial (SA) and atrioventricular (AV) nodes.[16] This added effect has enabled two agents (diltiazem and verapamil) to be useful in the treatment of various cardiac arrhythmias. The benzothiazepine derivative diltiazem has a more balanced effect between peripheral smooth muscle dilating properties of dihydropyridines and the myocardial depressing conduction effects of verapamil.

There still exists concern in both peer-reviewed literature as well as in clinical practice about deleterious cardiac effects of short-acting formulations of various CCBs.[17] As reported, short-acting nifedipine may increase the risk of adverse cardiovascular events and/or mortality.[1] Currently, the Joint National Committee on Prevention, Detection, Evaluation, and Treatment of High Blood Pressure (JNC 7) recommends the use of a long-acting nifedipine product such as Adalat® CC or Procardia XL® instead and does not include rapid-release nifedipine products in its list of available oral antihypertensive drugs.[2]

A recent case-control study showed that hypertensive patients who had suffered a myocardial infarction were more commonly being treated with a CCB than were those who had not had a myocardial infarction.[9] In the meantime, the long-acting preparations of diltiazem, verapamil, and nifedipine, as well as newer dihydropyridine compounds, should continue to be prescribed for hypertensive patients who have indications for their use such as angina.

Centrally Acting α-Agonists

The centrally acting α-agonists include clonidine, guanabenz, guanfacine, and methyldopa; they lower blood pressure by stimulating central α_2-receptors. It is believed that methyldopa, through its conversion to α-methylnorepinephrine, acts similarly to clonidine, guanabenz, and guanfacine by stimulation of α_2-receptors, causing a decrease in sympathetic outflow to the kidneys, heart, and peripheral vasculature.[1] The result is a decrease in

Table 5-4.

Comparison of Currently Available Oral β-adrenergic Receptor Blockers in the Treatment of Hypertension[2,3,6,7]

Drug	Usual Dose Range[†] Total mg/day (Frequency per Day)	Cardio-selectivity[††]	ISA[‡]	MSA[‡‡]	Lipophilicity	α-Blockade	Predominant Route of Elimination
Acebutolol	200–800 (1)	Yes	Yes	Yes	Weak	No	Renal
Atenolol	25–100 (1–2)	Yes	No	No	Weak	No	Renal
Betaxolol	5–20 (1)	Yes	No	No	High	No	Hepatic with <15% Renal
Bisoprolol	2.5–10 (1)	Yes	No	No	Moderate	No	50% Hepatic, 50% Renal
Carteolol	2.5–10 (1)	No	Yes	No	No	No	60% Renal
Carvedilol	6.25–50 (2)	No	No	No		Yes	Hepatic
Labetolol	200–1200 (2)	No	No	Yes	Weak	Yes	Hepatic
Metoprolol*	50–300 (1–2)	Yes	No	No	Moderate	No	Hepatic
Nadolol	40–320 (1)	No	No	No	Weak	No	Renal
Penbutolol	10–20 (1)	No	Yes	No		No	5% Renal
Pindolol	10–60 (2)	No	Yes	Yes	Moderate	No	Renal (40%) and Hepatic
Propranolol**	40–480 (1–2)	No	No	Yes	High	No	Hepatic
Timolol	20–60 (2)	No	No	No	Weak	No	Renal (20%) and Hepatic

[†]These doses may be different than those listed in the *Physicians' Desk Reference*, which may be consulted for further information.

[††]Relative to propranolol, agents possessing cardioselectivity have a greater tendency to occupy the β_1-receptor in the heart, rather than the β_2-receptor in the lungs. However, this tendency is dose-dependent and can be lost with increasing doses.

[‡]Intrinsic sympathomimetic activity (ISA) refers to those agents having the ability to release catecholamines and to maintain a satisfactory heart rate, which might reduce the development of bronchoconstriction and other direct acting β-blocking effects.

[‡‡]Membrane stabilizing affects (MSA) refers to those agents, which when given in doses exceeding therapeutic levels possess a quinidine-like or "local anesthetic" effect on the cardiac action potential, and are capable of inducing arrhythmias.

*Two products are available: a metoprolol tartrate product, which is relatively short-acting and is dosed in a twice daily manner, and a metoprolol succinate, which is a longer-acting product and is dosed on a once daily manner.

**Two products are available: a short-acting one, which is given twice daily, and a longer-acting product (Inderal LA), which is dosed in a once daily manner.

peripheral vascular resistance, decreased blood pressure, and decreased cardiac output.

Direct-Acting Vasodilators

The predominant effect of these agents is to cause vasodilation of arterioles with a resultant decrease in peripheral vascular resistance and is associated with little effect on the venous system (hydralazine and minoxidil).[1] A reflex increase in heart rate and cardiac output is associated with the direct-acting vasodilators and might be contraindicated in hypertensive patients with a history of ischemic heart disease.

Diuretics

Recent evidence demonstrates that the diuretics are the most effective class of drugs in the treatment of hypertension.[13] In the treatment of hypertension, the use of diuretics primarily involves the use of three different classes of agents: (1) thiazide and related diuretics such as hydrochlorothiazide, (2) loop diuretics such as furosemide, and (3) potassium-sparing diuretics such as spironolactone. In this section, each of these three classes will be covered separately to minimize confusion.

Thiazide and related diuretics consist of the largest class of diuretics used in the treatment of hypertension. Their primary mechanism of action is to increase the excretion of sodium (natriuretic ef-

Table 5-5.

Comparison of Currently Available Oral Calcium Channel Blockers in the Treatment of Hypertension[2,3,5,8,9]

Drug Class/Drug	Usual Dose Range[†] Total mg/day (Frequency per Day)	Elimination Characteristics/ Interactions	Drug–Food Interactions
Dihydropyridines		Metabolized to less active metabolites predominantly by cytochrome P-450 CYP3A. Inducers and inhibitors of biotransformation mechanism (i.e., rifampin, ketoconazole, cimetidine) can alter their metabolism, and vice versa.	Grapefruit juice, as an inhibitor of P-450 CYP3A biotransformation, down-regulates CYP3A and reduces first-pass metabolism, which increases peak serum levels and bioavailability.[‡]
Amlodipine	2.5–10 (1)		
Felodipine	2.5–20 (1)		
Isradipine	5–20 (1–2)[††]		
Nicardipine	60–90 (2)		
Nifedipine	30–120 (1)		
Nisoldipine	20–60 (1)		
Nondihydropyridines		Similar to dihydropyridines. Additionally, have been shown to inhibit P-glycoprotein-mediated drug transport which may alter intestinal absorption of other drugs (i.e., daunorubicin, epirubicin, idarubicin, paclitaxel). Combination of inhibition of CYP3A and P-glycoprotein increases bioavailability of cyclosporine, resulting in reduced dosing needs.	
Diltiazem	120–360 (1–2)[*]		
Verapamil	90–480 (2)[**]		
	120–480 (1)[**]		

[†]These doses may be different than those listed in the *Physicians' Desk Reference*, which may be used to obtain additional information.

[††]A short-acting product (DynaCirc) is available and requires two doses per day, and a longer-acting product (DynaCirc CR) is available and requires one dose per day.

[*]A short-acting product (Cardizem SR) is available and requires two doses per day, and a longer-acting product (Cardizem CD) is available and requires one dose per day.

[**]Short-acting products (Isoptin SR, Calan SR) are available and require two doses per day, and longer-acting products (Verelan, Covera HS) are available and require one dose per day.

[‡]Clinical trials have shown that one glass of grapefruit juice is able to significantly increase bioavailability and enhance blood pressure reduction, increase heart rate, and increase vasodilator effects.[8]

fect) and chloride by the kidneys through their ability to inhibit absorption within the cortical region of the distal convoluted tubule of the kidneys.[3] Thiazide diuretics create a mild diuresis, resulting in the excretion of potassium, bicarbonate, magnesium, and phosphate along with sodium and chloride and a reduction in the excretion of calcium. The primary clinical effects of thiazide diuretics in the treatment of hypertension occur due to the reduction in interstitial fluid volume, although other mechanisms such as reduced sensitivity of receptor sites to vasoconstrictive hormones, a direct dilating effect on peripheral vessels, and reduced concentrations of intracellular calcium due to reduced sodium concentrations have also been described.[1] Thiazide diuretics are normally considered the preferred diuretics for patients with hypertension. However, thiazide diuretics are not effective in patients with impaired renal function (creatinine clearance less than 30 ml/min), and alternative agents such as the loop diuretics are often used in such situations.

Diuretics have a direct relationship between the natriuretic response of the given agent and the amount of diuretic reaching the site of action, which determines the pharmacodynamics of the drug.[18] For each commercially available diuretic, there is a threshold quantity of drug that must be delivered to the site of action in order to create a pharmacologic response. Clinically, this requires the appropriate titration of each diuretic in each patient to determine the correct amount of drug that must be given to a specific patient to obtain appropriate concentrations at the site of action to elicit a diuretic response. For any given patient, the maximal effect by an individual diuretic is the same, so the choice of an agent within the class is primarily due to differing pharmacokinetic characteristics and costs.

Currently, based on available outcomes data, convenience, and cost of therapy, low-dose thiazide diuretic therapy appears to be the best first-line agents.[19] Thiazide diuretics have demonstrated the ability to lower blood pressure and reduce the risk of death, coronary artery disease, and stroke when compared to high-dose thiazide diuretics, β-blockers, CCBs, or ACE inhibitors.[11,19] Although there is growing evidence that blood pressure reduction alone might not be the ideal surrogate marker, until additional evidence becomes available to substantiate this belief, clinicians need to decide on a therapeutic regimen based on currently available evidence.

The ALLHAT blood pressure study was a randomized, double-blind trial.[12,15] It involved 42,418 participants ages 55 and older, and was conducted at 623 clinics and centers across the United States, Canada, Puerto Rico, and the U.S. Virgin Islands. Participants had hypertension (140/90 mm Hg or higher) and at least one other of the risk factors for heart disease, which include cigarette smoking and type 2 diabetes.[15] Participants were randomly assigned to receive one of four drugs: a diuretic (chlorthalidone), a CCB (amlodipine), an ACE inhibitor (lisinopril), and an α-adrenergic blocker (doxazosin). Subjects were followed on average for 4.9 years. They received additional antihypertensive drugs if their doctor thought it necessary to control their blood pressure.[15] As mentioned previously, the α-adrenergic blocker arm of the study was stopped in March 2000 because those on the drug had 25% more cardiovascular events and were twice as likely to be hospitalized for heart failure as users of the diuretic.

All three classes of drugs reported on including diuretics, CCBs, and ACE inhibitors have been previously shown to lower blood pressure and reduce cardiovascular complications. However, in head-to-head comparisons, the diuretics were shown to be superior in treating high blood pressure and preventing cardiovascular events.[15] As reported in the most recent report, after about 5 years of follow-up, compared to participants who were taking the diuretic, those on the CCB had the following effects:[13]

- On average, about a 1 mm Hg higher systolic blood pressure
- 38% higher risk of developing heart failure and 35% higher risk of being hospitalized for the condition

Additionally, compared to participants who were taking the diuretic, those on the ACE inhibitor had the following effects:[13]

- On average, about a 2 mm Hg higher systolic blood pressure and 4 mm Hg higher in African-Americans
- 15% higher risk of stroke
- 40% higher risk of stroke for African-Americans
- 19% higher risk of developing heart failure
- 11% greater risk of being hospitalized or treated for angina (chest pain)
- 10% greater risk of having to undergo a coronary revascularization (such as coronary artery bypass surgery)

An important take-home message from the study was that with the publication of the ALLHAT findings, the evidence would suggest that drug treatment for high blood pressure should begin with a diuretic, which can be tolerated by a large majority of patients.[2,13] However, for those who cannot tolerate a diuretic, an ACE inhibitor, CCB, or a beta-blocker may be used to start treatment.

Loop diuretics work within the thick ascending limb of Henle's loop where they have a potent natriuretic effect and reduce the reabsorption of sodium by blocking the sodium–potassium–chloride transporter.[1] Loop diuretics increase the rate of delivery of fluid and electrolytes within the renal tubule to the more distal sites of hydrogen and potassium secretion into the tubules. The four loop diuretics, bumetanide, ethacrynic acid, torsemide, and furosemide, cause a contraction in the plasma volume, which results in the stimulation of aldosterone from the adrenal cortex.[1] The effect of aldosterone on the kidneys is responsible for the reabsorption of sodium in the distal tubule and the resultant loss of hydrogen and potassium ions in exchange for sodium.[1] The loop diuretics are considered the most potent of the diuretics (based on sodium and water excretion), and lower blood pressure by reducing plasma and extracellular fluid volume, which is initially accompanied by a reduction in cardiac output. Over time, cardiac output returns toward normal and is accompanied by a reduction in peripheral vascular resistance.[1]

Loop diuretics are not routinely considered in the treatment of hypertension, although they have shown benefit in heart failure and other cardiac syndromes. Loop diuretics are frequently used as alternatives in patients who are either refractory to thiazide diuretics or patients with declining renal function who are unable to receive thiazide diuretics.

Potassium-sparing diuretics work in the distal convoluted tubule of the kidneys by preventing some of the sodium exchange for potassium that occurs in this part of the nephron.[1] Due to their very weak diuretic effect and antihypertensive effects, these agents are not routinely used as antihypertensive agents. They have, however, been used in conjunction with thiazide diuretics to reduce potassium loss or correct hypokalemia. There is the potential for hyperkalemia when the agents are used in conjunction with ACE inhibitors. The currently available agents amiloride, spironolactone, eplerenone, and triamterene demonstrate the same therapeutic effect, but amiloride and triamterene act directly on the distal tubule to reduce sodium and water reabsorption, while spironolactone and eplerenone work directly on aldosterone-binding sites to reduce sodium and water reabsorption.[1]

Patients who have demonstrated allergies to sulfonamides might demonstrate cross-sensitivity to all thiazides, bumetanide, torsemide, and furosemide. Ethacrynic acid would prove to be a therapeutic alternative as a nonsulfonamide loop diuretic.

Postganglionic Adrenergic Neuron Blockers

Reserpine is a rauwolfia alkaloid available in the treatment of hypertension; currently, however, the rauwolfia alkaloids are used infrequently.[1] Reserpine works at the postganglionic neurons of the sympathetic nervous system by depleting the concentration of catecholamines (norepinephrine and epinephrine) and serotonin. This results in reduced sympathetic actions with a resultant decrease in cardiac output and peripheral vascular resistance. Rauwolfia alkaloids are considered relatively weak antihypertensive agents, and in many patients there is the need to add other agents to the regimen in order to cause the desired therapeutic effect. Diuretics are often added to regimens to reduce the degree of sodium and water retention secondary to the use of reserpine.

Much attention has been given in the past to the significant side effects associated with the use of reserpine in high doses. Mental depression is of particular concern to the elderly hypertensive patient who might be placed on reserpine. The elderly appear to be more prone to depression than younger patients. Mental depression had previously received much attention due to the potential suicidal effects reported from reserpine, which has probably resulted in a drastic reduction in the clinical use of this class of drugs in the treatment of mild-to-moderate hypertension. Today, small doses are known to be effective, well tolerated, and very inexpensive.

Summary

The JNC 7 guidelines provide a reference point for initiating drug therapy for patients with hypertension as well as a rational treatment algorithm, which allows clinicians to design individual therapeutic regimens for patients based on the individual characteristics for each patient.[2] A pharmacist's ability to understand the different mechanisms of action for the various classes of antihypertensive agents provides an excellent opportunity to actively participate on the health care team by designing antihypertensive regimens, which contribute favorably to a patient's care. The initiation of patient therapeutic regimens requires an appreciation for the different mechanisms of action among different antihypertensives as well as their associated side effect profiles. Due to the major role which the relationship between mechanisms of action for antihypertensives and patient comorbidities have on drug selection, the pharmacist who is able to apply pharmacological principles will be better suited to designing therapeutic regimens for hypertensive patients and will provide significant value as a member of the antihypertensive health care team.

Key Points for Patients

- The treatment of hypertension is a life-long process and requires active participation by the patient if it is to be successful.
- There are many medications available to treat hypertension, but a patient's prescription is specific to him or her, based on many specific findings about hypertension and comorbidities.
- It is important for patients to know the names of their medications, how often to take the medications, and what are the key side effects.
- If a patient's treatment is confusing, he or she should make sure to follow-up with a health care provider to explain and monitor the antihypertensive regimen.

References

1. USP DI 2001 21st ed. Drug information for the health care professional, vol. 1. Englewood: Micromedex; 2001:1266–73.

2. The seventh report of the Joint National Committee on Prevention, Detection, Evaluation, and Treatment of High Blood Pressure. The JNC 7 report. *JAMA.* 2003; 289:2560–72.

3. Handbook of clinical drug data. 9th ed. Anderson PO, Knoben JE, Troutman WG, eds. Stamford, CT: Appleton & Lange; 1999:314–60, 670–86.

4. Carretero OA, Oparil S. Essential hypertension: part II: treatment. *Circulation.* 2000; 101(4):446–53.

5. Abernethy DR, Schwartz JB. Drug therapy: calcium-antagonist drugs. *N Engl J Med.* 1999; 341:1447–57.

6. Weibert RT. In: Textbook of therapeutics: drug and disease management. 7th ed. Herfindal ET, Gourley DR, eds. Baltimore: Lippincott Williams & Wilkins; 2000.

7. Frishman WH. In: Clinical essays on the heart. vol. 2. Hurst JW, ed. New York: McGraw-Hill, 1983:25–63.

8. Kane GC, Lipsky JJ. Drug-grapefruit juice interactions. *Mayo Clinic Proceedings.* 2000; 75:933–42.

9. Abernethy DR, Flockhart DA. Molecular basis of cardiovascular drug metabolism: implications for predicting clinically important drug interactions. *Circulation.* 2000; 101:1749–53.

10. Brown NJ, Vaughan DE. Angiotensin-converting enzyme inhibitors. *Circulation.* 1998; 97:1411–20.

11. Schoolwerth AC, Sica DA, Ballermann BJ et al. Renal considerations in angiotensin converting enzyme inhibitor therapy: a statement for healthcare professionals from the Council on the Kidney in Cardiovascular Disease and the Council for High Blood Pressure Research of the American Heart Association [American Heart Association scientific statement]. *Circulation.* 2001; 104:1985–91.

12. Bicket DP. Using ACE inhibitors appropriately. *Am Fam Physician.* 2002; 66:461–8.

13. The ALLHAT Officers and Coordinators for the ALLHAT Collaborative Research Group. Major outcomes in high-risk hypertensive patients randomized to angiotensin-converting enzyme inhibitor or calcium channel blocker vs diuretic: the Antihypertensive and Lipid-Lowering Treatment to Prevent Heart Attack Trial (ALLHAT). *JAMA.* 2002; 288:2981–97.

14. Burnier M. Angiotensin II type 1 receptor blockers. *Circulation.* 2001; 103(6):904–12.

15. Major cardiovascular events in hypertensive patients randomized to doxazosin vs chlorthalidone: the Antihypertensive and Lipid-Lowering Treatment to Prevent Heart Attack Trial (ALLHAT). ALLHAT Collaborative Research Group. *JAMA.* 2000; 283:1967–75.

16. Kaplan NM, Gifford RW Jr. Choice of initial therapy for hypertension. *JAMA.* 1996; 275(20):1577–80.

17. Psaty BM, Heckbert SR, Koepsell TD et al. The risk of myocardial infarction associated with antihypertensive drug therapies. *JAMA.* 1995; 274:620–5.

18. Brater DC. Diuretic therapy. *N Engl J Med.* 1998; 339:387–95.

19. Chobanian AV, Bakris GL, Black HR et al. Seventh report of the Joint National Committee on Prevention, Detection, Evaluation, and Treatment of High Blood Pressure. JNC-complete version. *Hypertension.* 2003; 42:1206–52.

Chapter 6:

Initiation of Therapy

Jacqueline D. Joss and Beth Bryles Phillips

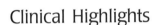

Clinical Highlights

- What evidence supports that lifestyle modification, including weight loss, exercise, sodium restriction, and moderation of alcohol intake, is essential in the avoidance and treatment of hypertension?
- Which antihypertensive agents are appropriate for initial therapy in a patient with uncomplicated hypertension?
- How do age, sex, and race affect the choice of antihypertensive drug therapy?
- What types of concomitant medical conditions affect antihypertensive drug therapy decisions?
- What types of patient-related factors may affect the choice of antihypertensive drug therapy?

The risk of cardiovascular disease depends both on the level of blood pressure elevation and the presence of other cardiovascular risk factors or target organ damage. For these reasons, the seventh report of the Joint National Committee on Prevention, Detection, Evaluation, and Treatment of High Blood Pressure has based the initial treatment guidelines (JNC 7) on the actual presenting blood pressure and presence or absence of these risk factors (**Table 6-1**).[1] Patients with prehypertension should be encouraged to begin lifestyle modification to minimize progression to hypertension. Patients with hypertension must be counseled on appropriate lifestyle modification, in addition to initiating drug therapy. Patients with stage 1 hypertension are to be started on single drug therapy. Patients with more advanced (stage 2) hypertension should be considered for initial dual antihypertensive therapy, since it is unlikely that target blood pressures will be achieved using one agent alone. This chapter will serve to outline the lifestyle modifications and the process of drug therapy selection that should be applied to all patients with hypertension.

Nonpharmacologic Therapy

Lifestyle modification, which includes weight loss, regular aerobic exercise, reduction of salt intake, moderation of alcohol use, and smoking cessation, is the cornerstone in the treatment of hypertension. Following the Dietary Approach to Stop

Hypertension (DASH) eating plan, which is a diet rich in fruits, vegetables, and low-fat calcium while minimizing dietary saturated and total fat, is another important component of adjusting one's lifestyle to improve blood pressure. Each individual intervention has been shown to have beneficial effects on blood pressure, which will be reviewed in this chapter.

A combination of interventions was studied in the PREMIER trial.[2] This study was a good study of "real life" intervention, since patients purchased their own food, rather than being supplied with prepared meals as in the DASH trial (discussed later in this chapter).[3] In PREMIER, the "advice only" group of patients received a single 30-minute session with a dietitian, who discussed nonpharmacologic factors that affect blood pressure (weight, sodium intake, physical activity, and the DASH diet). The other two groups received more intense counseling during 14 group meetings and four individual sessions over the 6-month study period. In addition, one of the two latter groups received more specific counseling on the DASH diet. Both of these two groups were asked to keep food diaries to document their modification of lifestyle. The data revealed that all three groups had a significant decrease in blood pressure. While the individual interventions did not demonstrate an additive effect on blood pressure lowering, each additional intervention did demonstrate further improvement. The trial also demonstrated that even one-time counseling on lifestyle modification has a beneficial effect on blood pressure. This is useful information

Table 6-1.
Classification and Management of Blood Pressure for Adults*[5]

BP Classification	SBP mm Hg	DBP mm Hg	Lifestyle Modification	Initial Drug Therapy	
				Without Compelling Indication	With Compelling Indications
Normal	<120	and <80	Encourage	No antihypertensive drug indicated.	Drug(s) for compelling indications.[‡]
Prehypertension	120–139	or 80–89	Yes		
Stage 1 hypertension	140–159	or 90–99	Yes	Thiazide-type diuretics for most. May consider ACE I, ARB, BB, CCB, or combination.	Drug(s) for the compelling indications.[‡] Other antihypertensive drugs (diuretics, ACE I, ARB, BB, CCB) as needed.
Stage 2 hypertension	≥160	or ≥100	Yes	Two-drug combination for most[†] (usually thiazide-type diuretic and ACE I or ARB or BB or CCB).	

*Treatment determined by highest BP category.

ACE I = angiotensin-converting-enzyme inhibitor; ARB = angiotensin receptor blocker; BB = beta-blocker; CCB = calcium channel blocker; DBP = diastolic blood pressure; SBP = systolic blood pressure.

[†]Initial combined therapy should be used cautiously in those at risk for orthostatic hypotension.

[‡]Treat patients with chronic kidney disease or diabetes to BP goal of <130/80 mm Hg.

(Reprinted with permission from the seventh report of the Joint National Committee on Prevention, Detection, Evaluation, and Treatment of High Blood Pressure. National Heart, Lung, and Blood Institute, National Institutes of Health, May 2003; NIH publication no. 03-5233.)

since time constraints in busy clinic practices do not always allow for intense dietary counseling. Clinicians should, however, attempt to emphasize these lifestyle modifications at subsequent visits, even after drug therapy has been initiated.

Weight Reduction

In the United States, obesity has become a major health hazard. The prevalence of obesity in the United States had risen from 25% in the late 1980s to 33% in the early 1990s as determined by NHANES III.[4] According to this alarming trend, the surgeon general had predicted that 40% of the U.S. population was obese in the year 2000.

Epidemiological studies support a positive correlation between blood pressure and body weight.[5] More recent studies confirm that excess body weight, as demonstrated by an elevated body mass index (BMI), is directly associated with elevated blood pressure.[6] A BMI of 26–28 kg/m^2 can increase the risk of high blood pressure by up to 180% when compared with a BMI of 23 or less. Besides BMI, the type of obesity is also important in the incidence of hypertension. Android (abdominal) obesity is associated with a greater incidence of hypertension, when compared with gynoid or "pear

shaped" obesity, which is an accumulation of fat in the gluteofemoral area.[7] Obesity is also a risk factor for dyslipidemia, diabetes mellitus, and cardiovascular mortality.[8,9]

There are several proposed mechanisms by which excess body weight can elevate blood pressure. An elevated BMI results in increased plasma volume and cardiac output, resulting in elevated blood pressure. This theory is supported by the fact that both these variables can be decreased by weight loss even if the sodium intake is kept constant.[10] Another proposed mechanism is a decrease in renal filtration surface, which leads to sodium retention.[11] Obesity leads to insulin resistance and hyperinsulinemia, which can increase tubular reabsorption of sodium and increase sympathetic nervous system activity.[12]

A BMI of 25 is generally considered a reasonable upper limit of healthy weight. The International Obesity Taskforce has provided a more detailed classification of weight by BMI (**Table 6-2**).[13]

Patients with hypertension should be prescribed an individualized weight reduction program of reduced calorie intake and exercise. It is important to note that even a moderate amount of weight loss can have a significant effect on blood pressure. The World Health Organization (WHO) recommends

Table 6-2.
World Health Organization Obesity Classification

WHO Obesity Classification (Geneva 1998)	BMI, kg/m²
Healthy weight	18.5–24.9
Overweight	25–29.9
Class I obesity	30–34.9
Class II obesity	35–39.9
Class III obesity	40.0 or higher

that the practitioner recommend an initial weight loss of 5 kg, with subsequent 5-kg increments to be attempted later, depending on the patient's initial weight.[14] A 6-month study of patients with high-normal blood pressure at baseline, who were at 110–165% of their desirable body weight, showed that a 4.3-kg weight loss resulted in a significant reduction in both systolic and diastolic blood pressure.[15] This study demonstrated that even though the weight loss and decrease in blood pressure were difficult to maintain in the long term (36 months), there was a reduction in the progression from high-normal blood pressure to hypertension in patients assigned to weight loss intervention. In overweight patients with existing hypertension, a 3.5-kg weight loss allowed for a 30% reduction in the need for anti-hypertensive medication.[16] Besides enhancing the effect of antihypertensive medications, this moderate weight reduction can also significantly decrease the incidence of other known cardiovascular risk factors such as hyperlipidemia and diabetes.[17]

The key to weight loss, and thereby control of cardiovascular risk factors, is a commitment to ongoing lifestyle modifications. Many patients require an enrollment in a formal dietary program. This may be essential in patients with a limited knowledge of appropriate nutrition. The behavioral treatment approach to weight loss helps patients develop better eating and exercise habits essential in maintaining weight loss.[18] While exercise may not necessarily increase the initial weight loss with calorie reduction, it is an important factor in helping to maintain the weight loss in the long term.[19]

"Fad" diets and diets that recommend a particular diet composition (e.g., low carbohydrate, high protein) have generally been discouraged, since they do not produce a greater weight loss than a reduced calorie, low-fat diet.[20] In addition, these diets often

do not follow the American Heart Association guidelines for reduced fat intake.[21]

The low-carbohydrate diets recently have come into the spotlight again with the release of two randomized trials investigating the weight loss and effect on cholesterol by these diets. A 1-year study of the Atkins diet was conducted in 63 moderately obese patients (BMI 34).[22] The Atkins diet (low carbohydrate, high protein, high fat) resulted in a significantly greater weight loss at 3 and 6 months when compared with the conventional diet of low calorie, high carbohydrate, and low fat (−7.0±6.5% versus −3.2±5.6% of body weight at 6 months). The difference, however, became nonsignificant at 12 months. The Atkins diet produced a greater increase in high-density lipoprotein (HDL) cholesterol and a greater decrease in triglycerides. A similar 6-month trial of a low-carbohydrate versus low-fat and low-calorie diet in 132 severely obese patients (BMI 43) had a similar result. Weight loss was greater at 6 months with the low-carbohydrate diet (−5.8±8.6 kg versus −1.9±4.2 kg).[23] The triglyceride reductions were greater in the low-carbohydrate diet, and nondiabetics on a low-carbohydrate diet had an improvement in insulin sensitivity.

Despite these positive results, readers should be aware that there were shortcomings to the trials. The studies did not demonstrate a long-term superiority of the low-carbohydrate diet, as evidenced by the nonsignificant difference at 1 year. The overall absolute magnitude of weight loss difference was relatively small (4 kg) and adherence in both diet groups was low. A review of the efficacy and safety of low-carbohydrate studies confirmed that there is very little data on long-term effects of these diets and that weight loss is generally associated with the restriction of calories rather than the carbohydrate intake per se.[24] The positive effect on lipid levels should also be viewed with caution. While low-carbohydrate diets do generally reduce triglycerides, the rise in HDL may be related to a change in HDL subfractions that occurs with an increase of saturated fats, and this change may not be beneficial. More research to investigate this issue may be required. Other diets that promote severe caloric restriction may increase initial weight loss; however, they generally do not increase the long-term success of maintaining weight loss.[25]

Weight-loss medications, such as phentermine and sibutramine, are generally not recommended because many of these agents will elevate blood pressure and many of them are not approved for

Figure 6-1.
Evidence-Based Algorithm for the Treatment of Obesity

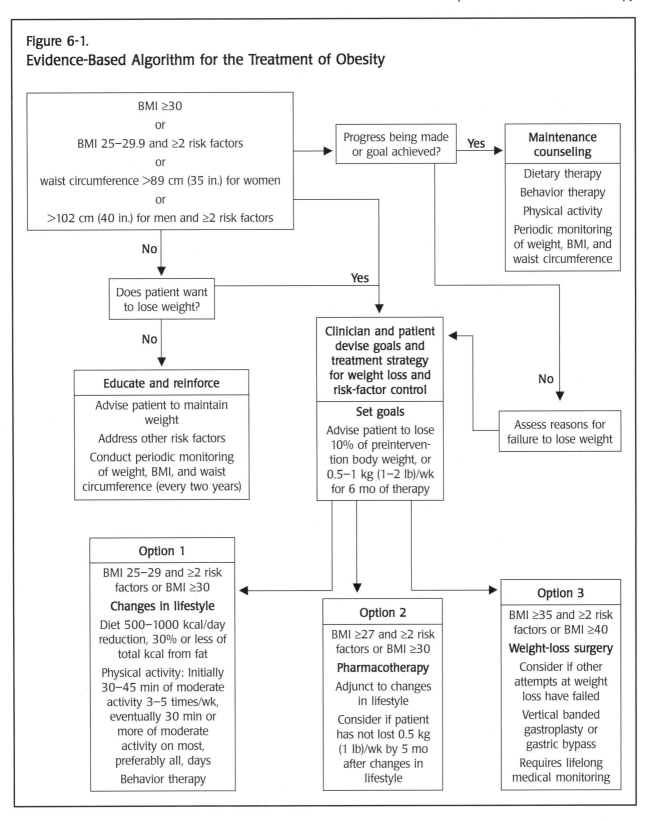

(Reprinted with permission from *N Engl J Med.* 2002; 346:591–602.)

long-term use.[26] These agents should be reserved for patients who are at a substantial increased risk and should only be used as an adjunct to behavioral therapy. **Figure 6-1** outlines an evidence-based algorithm for the treatment of obesity as recommended by the National Institutes of Health.[26]

The DASH Eating Plan

The DASH diet promotes a diet rich in fruits, vegetables, and low-fat dairy products, while reducing the amount of saturated and total fat. It has been shown that strict application of the DASH diet can reduce blood pressure as much as some drugs (11.4/5.5 mm Hg) in hypertensive patients.[3] This dietary modification provides benefits extending beyond blood pressure lowering (e.g., diabetes mellitus, hyperlipidemia) and should be recommended to all persons with or without hypertension.

Physical Activity

A sedentary lifestyle is a risk factor for cardiovascular disease and it has been estimated that patients are at a 30–50% greater risk of developing hypertension if they do not participate in regular physical exercise.[27] Regular aerobic exercise is not only essential in the maintenance of weight loss,[19] but it is also an important factor in controlling blood pressure independent of the change in body weight associated with exercise.[28] Aerobic exercise will decrease blood pressure even in participants whose BMI is within the normal range. Studies of the effect of exercise on weight loss have shown that blood pressure is significantly reduced, even when the patients did not lose weight. The underlying mechanism of this effect may be related to the reduction in insulin resistance and insulin levels by aerobic exercise.[29] Higher insulin levels have been associated with an increased risk of hypertension due to effects on the sympathetic nervous system and renal excretion of sodium.[12]

Patients should be encouraged to increase their activity to include at least 30–45 minutes of brisk walking on most days of the week.[30] The objective of a conditioning program is to reach an exercise level at which the body is achieving about 70% of maximal predicted oxygen uptake, a level that is attained when the heart rate reaches approximately 80% of the maximal predicted rate. This rate is approximately 170 beats per minute (bpm) for 20–29-year-olds, decreasing by 10 bpm for every decade in age to 130 for 60–69-year-olds.[31] Optimal

conditioning in healthy persons occurs with aerobic activity at the target heart rate for 20 minutes at least three times a week. Even low-intensity exercise which does not result in conditioning will result in some health benefits; however, for exercise to result in an improvement in physical fitness, the muscles and the organ system must be exercised at a greater intensity than the level the person is accustomed to. The overload must be applied gradually for maximal effectiveness and safety. Patients with cardiac conditions should consult their physician, since they may require an initial cardiac stress test or referral to a specialist or medically supervised exercise program. Patients over 35 years of age and those with major risk factors for atherosclerosis should have a resting ECG and physical examination. Nondiagnostic fitness tests for apparently healthy individuals are usually available at health clubs and wellness centers for a nominal fee.

Moderation of Sodium Intake

Epidemiologic evidence has shown that there is an association between high sodium intake and elevated blood pressure.[32] In addition, certain subgroups of the population appear to be more sensitive to changes in dietary sodium intake, with African-American, elderly, and obese patients having the most significant response in blood pressure.[33] The importance of sodium restriction in the treatment of hypertension was verified in a recent report of the DASH trial.[34] Varying levels of sodium intake (3.5, 2.3, or 1.2 grams per day) were studied in persons with or without hypertension. The subjects were also randomly assigned to a control diet typical of intake in the United States or the DASH diet, which is rich in vegetables, fruit, whole grains, poultry, fish, and low-fat dairy products. Blood pressure was significantly reduced by decreasing dietary sodium intake in hypertensive and normotensive subjects in both diet groups. While both interventions lowered blood pressure significantly, the combination had greater effects than either intervention alone. Subjects with hypertension on the low-sodium and DASH diets had an 11.5 mm Hg lowering in systolic blood pressure. The response in blood pressure lowering was also greater with the more sodium-restricted diet when compared with small reductions in salt intake. These results confirm the recommendations by the JNC 7 guidelines that patients should follow the DASH diet and reduce sodium intake to less than 2.4 grams of sodium (6 grams of sodium chloride) per day. It has been estimated that the common diet in the United States currently amounts to 6–9 grams of sodium per day. Indicators of a high-salt diet include:

- prepared foods such as frozen dinners, packaged goods, and processed meats and cheese
- salty foods such as potato chips, salted nuts, and pretzels
- eating in restaurants frequently
- using salt at the table

Most salt consumed by Americans is the result of the frequent use of processed foods, and about 25% of total salt consumed occurs as a result of adding salt at the table.[35] By encouraging the intake of fresh fruits and vegetables, avoiding processed foods, and by not having a saltshaker at the table, most people should be able to maintain a sodium intake of less than 2.4 grams per day. In the DASH trial, food was controlled and supplied to participants allowing the detailed evaluation of dietary effects on blood pressure. The lowest level of sodium intake studied in this trial of 1.2 grams per day cannot realistically be achieved by most Americans without a major change in their lifestyle. Salt substitutes can be utilized to decrease sodium intake. Since most salt substitutes contain potassium chloride, potassium levels must be monitored in patients with renal dysfunction and in patients taking potassium-sparing diuretics, angiotensin II receptor antagonists, and ACE inhibitors or aldosterone antagonists. An occasionally unrecognized source of sodium is baking soda, which may be used by some patients as an antacid. Even a teaspoon of baking soda contains a significant amount of sodium. Patients with hypertension as well as patients who need to practice sodium restriction for other reasons (e.g., heart failure) should be counseled to avoid baking soda.

Potassium Intake

The importance of potassium in the control of hypertension is unclear. The Intersalt study showed that, while blood pressure was directly related to sodium intake, it was also inversely related to potassium intake.[36] In this study, potassium intake was judged by 24-hour urinary potassium excretion. It was determined that a 30–45-mmol increase in potassium was associated with a 2–3-mm Hg decrease in systolic blood pressure. The DASH trial verified that the effect of potassium is independent and in addition to the effect of the sodium reduction.[3,34] Potassium increased from 37 mmol/day to 71 mmol/day by increasing fruit and vegetable consumption, and blood pressure was still significantly reduced even when sodium intake was kept at a same low level. Clinical trials using potassium chloride have shown a similar decrease in blood pressure when compared to the dietary potassium in fruits and vegetables.[37] It is, however, preferred that the population increases potassium intake by eating more fruits and vegetables because of the overall beneficial effect of this intervention on health. Patients on diuretic therapy should be closely monitored for the need of potassium supplements.

Calcium Intake

Hypertension is more prevalent in geographic areas supplied with "soft" water, i.e., water that contains a limited amount of calcium. Population data indicate that dietary calcium intake is inversely related to the likelihood of becoming hypertensive.[38,39] The overall effect of calcium supplementation on lowering blood pressure is minimal; therefore, calcium supplementation for this purpose is not currently recommended,[40] although patients should maintain an adequate intake for the prevention of osteoporosis.

Moderation of Alcohol Intake

Moderate intake of alcohol may be cardioprotective. One epidemiological study demonstrated a lower overall mortality rate in individuals who drank one or two drinks per day when compared to nondrinkers.[41] The overall death rate was lowest in those consuming one drink per day. The study included mostly middle-aged and elderly middle-class people, thereby excluding higher risk groups such as binge-drinkers, members of lower socioeconomic groups, and populations in which deaths from accidents, violence, and other external causes outnumber the deaths from cardiovascular events. It is known that there is an increased risk of accidents, violence, and several types of cancer at all levels of alcohol consumption above zero.[42,43] It should, therefore, not be recommended to nondrinkers to begin drinking alcohol for cardioprotection.

Hypertension incidence and severity have been linked to excessive alcohol intake.[44] The effect of alcohol on blood pressure increases with age. It is independent of the type of beverage consumed and additive to the effect of being overweight, using contraceptives, and having a high-salt diet.[45] It has been estimated that alcohol is a causal or contributing factor to the incidence of hypertension in 11% of all men.[46] Alcohol decreases the effectiveness of antihypertensive medications, but this effect is usually reversible within a few weeks of reduced intake.[47] Heavy drinkers (five or more standard drinks per day) may have a transient rise in blood pressure during acute alcohol withdrawal.

If patients consume alcohol, they should be counseled to limit their alcohol intake to no more than two drinks of alcohol per day (1 ounce or 30 ml of ethanol). This amount of alcohol is contained in 24 ounces of beer, 10 ounces of wine, or 2 ounces of 100-proof whisky. It is recommended that women limit their alcohol to half this amount, since they absorb more alcohol than men due to a decrease in gastric alcohol dehydrogenase activity and decreased first-pass metabolism.[48] Lighter weight persons also should abide by the lower intake because of an increased susceptibility to the effects of alcohol. Another factor to consider is that alcohol is a concentrated source of calories and has no nutritional value. Reducing alcohol intake may help with weight loss and reduce triglyceride levels.

Smoking Cessation

Cigarette smoking is known to be a powerful risk factor for coronary heart disease, stroke, peripheral vascular disease, and other cardiovascular disorders. Smoking cessation should be strongly recommended in all patients, including those with hypertension, to reduce the risk of mortality. A review of all smoking cessation trials in patients with coronary heart disease confirmed a risk reduction of overall mortality by more than one-third by this intervention.[49]

It is controversial whether smoking should be considered a contributing factor in the development of sustained hypertension. The controversy arises from studies that have actually shown an increase in clinic blood pressure after smoking cessation.[50] It has been postulated that former smokers may have higher blood pressure than never smokers, because of a higher prevalence of overweight and obese subjects in this group.[51] The same study did, however, show that current smoking men were at greater risk for hypertension than those who have never smoked, which was independent of body weight. Ambulatory blood pressure monitoring has demonstrated that smoking cessation decreased daytime systolic blood pressure and heart rate significantly in postmenopausal women, presumably due to reduced sympathetic activity.[52] Interestingly, these effects were not noted through clinic blood pressure measurements. Other authors have confirmed that smokers frequently have higher 24-hour ambulatory blood pressures than nonsmokers, even if office visit readings are the same or even lower in smokers.[53]

Overall, the evidence suggests that besides being a risk factor for cardiovascular disease, smoking contributes to the maintenance of high blood pressure. Patients who smoke will decrease the amount of protection they will obtain from their antihypertensive medication.[54] It is imperative that health care providers stress smoking cessation at every encounter with the patient. Smoking cessation aids contain lower doses of nicotine and will therefore not elevate blood pressure.[55] Numerous resources are available to the clinician to help educate patients on smoking cessation (**Table 6-3**). Appendix 6-1 lists examples of smoking cessation websites. The U.S. Public Health Service has published detailed guidelines on the treatment of tobacco use and dependence (**Tables 6-4 – 6-7**).[56] In addition, brochures instructing the patient on the proper use of smoking cessation aids as well as phone numbers for the nearest smoking cessation class should always be kept on hand.

Caffeine Intake

According to the guidelines issued by JNC 6, there is no direct relationship between caffeine intake and the risk of developing hypertension. This has been confirmed by more recent studies. One cohort of 1017 normotensive men followed over 33 years found that drinking one cup of coffee a day was

Table 6-3.
Smoking Cessation Resources for Health Care Professionals and Patients

Agency for Health Care Policy and Research
  1-800-358-9295

American Pharmacists Association
  1-800-878-0729

Smoking, Tobacco, and Health Information Line
  1-800-232-1311

American Cancer Society
  1-800-ACS-2345

American Lung Association
  1-800-LUNG-USA

Table 6-4.

Strategies* to Assist Patients Willing To Quit Tobacco Use: the "5 As"

Action	Strategies for Implementation
Ask Implement an officewide system that ensures that tobacco use status is queried and documented for every patient at every clinic visit. Options include expanding vital signs to include tobacco status (see example) or to place tobacco use status stickers on all charts. Alternatively, computer reminder systems may be used.	Example: Expand the vital signs to include tobacco use. *Vital signs* *Blood pressure:_____Pulse:_____* *Weight:_____ Temp:_____* *Respiratory Rate:_____* *Tobacco use: current former never (circle one)*
Advise In a clear, strong, and personalized manner, urge every tobacco user to quit.	Advice should be: Clear: I think it is important for you to quit smoking now and I can help you. Strong: As your clinician, I need you to know that quitting smoking now is the most important thing you can do for your health now and in the future. Personalized: Explain the effect of tobacco on current health and the effect of tobacco use on children and others in the household.
Assess Determine willingness to make a quit attempt in the next 30 days	• If the patient is willing to quit, provide assistance. • If the patient is unwilling to quit, provide a motivational intervention. • If the patient is part of a special population (e.g., pregnant smoker, adolescent, racial minority), provide additional information.
Assist Aid the patient in quitting	• Help the patient with a quit plan. • Set a quit date. • Tell friends and coworkers about the plan and request support. • Anticipate challenges (nicotine-withdrawal symptoms). • Remove tobacco products from environment. • Provide practical counseling (e.g., also consider abstinence from alcohol, because alcohol use frequently causes relapse). • Provide social support from the office staff (be available for assistance) and help the patient to obtain social support at home and at work (ask your family/coworkers to support you). • Recommend the use of pharmacotherapy. • Prove supplementary materials available from federal agencies (e.g., www.ahrq.gov).
Arrange Schedule follow-up	• Timing: follow up should occur within a week of the quit date. A second follow-up should occur within the first month. • During follow-up, congratulate on success. If the patient has relapsed, review circumstances of relapse, and remind patient that a relapse should be viewed as a learning experience. Identify solutions for similar challenges in the future. Consider referral to more intensive treatment.

*Fiore MC, Bailey WC, Cohen SJ et al. Treating tobacco use and dependence. Quick reference guide for clinicians. Rockville, MD: U.S. Department of Health and Human Services. Public Health Service. October 2000. (No reprint permission necessary)

Table 6-5.
Enhancing Motivation To Quit Tobacco Use: the "5Rs" for the Patient Unwilling To Quit at this Time*

Relevance

Encourage the patient; explain why quitting is personally relevant. Motivational information has the greatest impact if it is relevant to the patient's disease status, family, or social situation (e.g., having children in the home, financial impact of smoking cessation).

Risks

The clinician should discuss the risks of tobacco use.

- Acute risks: asthma exacerbation, shortness of breath, harm to pregnancy, impotence, infertility
- Long-term risks: myocardial infarction, stroke, cancer, chronic obstructive pulmonary disease
- Environmental risks: risk of cancer and heart disease in spouse, increased risk of sudden infant death syndrome

Rewards

The clinician should ask the patient to identify benefits of stopping tobacco use.

- Improved health
- Improved taste of food
- Improved sense of smell
- Saving money
- Home, car, breath will smell better
- Setting a good example for children
- Have healthier babies and children
- Reduced aging and wrinkling of skin

Roadblocks

The clinician should ask the patient to identify barriers and note elements of treatment (i.e., pharmacotherapy, problem solving) that could address these barriers. Typical examples include:

- Withdrawal symptoms
- Weight gain
- Depression
- Enjoyment of tobacco

Repetition

The motivational intervention should be repeated every time an unmotivated patient visits the clinic setting. Tobacco users who have failed previous attempts to quit should be told that most people make repeated quit attempts before they are successful.

*Fiore MC, Bailey WC, Cohen SJ et al. Treating tobacco use and dependence. Quick reference guide for clinicians. Rockville, MD: U.S. Department of Health and Human Services. Public Health Service. October 2000. (No reprint permission necessary)

associated with a small increase in blood pressure; however, long-term coffee drinking did not increase the risk of developing hypertension.[57] In patients who drank five or more cups of coffee per day, the relative risk of hypertension was increased; however, this association became nonsignificant after adjustment for family history, BMI, smoking status, alcohol intake, and physical activity.

It is, however, known that caffeine acutely increases blood pressure, which has lead to the recommendation that patients should refrain from ingesting caffeine for 30 minutes prior to evaluation. A more recent investigation of the effects of acute caffeine intake demonstrated that patients with hypertension may, however, need to refrain for an even longer time before their blood pressure is checked.[58] In this study, an equivalent of two to three cups of coffee was given to subjects whose blood pressure ranged from the normotensive range to diagnosed hypertension. It was determined that the higher the blood pressure was at baseline, the more of an increase was seen up to an hour after caffeine intake. It is generally believed that tolerance develops to the acute pressor effect of caffeine; however, the data on this issue are contradictory. One investigation randomized normotensive and hypertensive individuals to abstinence from caffeine-containing drinks or five cups of caffeine-containing coffee per day after a 2-week washout period.[59] In normotensive subjects, the blood pressure did not increase after 2 weeks. However, in hypertensive individuals, 24-hour blood pressure was significantly increased by caffeine (4.8/3.0 mm Hg, p<0.05).

It has been postulated that regular coffee use may be harmful to some hypertensive patients for reasons that are not clearly established yet. Some investigators have proposed a higher sensitivity to the cardiovascular effects of caffeine due to a genetic susceptibility to hypertension. More studies are needed to clarify this issue. In the meantime, it seems prudent to suggest reduced caffeine intake in patients who are severely hypertensive or in patients whose blood pressure is difficult to control. A trial off caffeine with close follow-up of the blood pressure may be an option in certain patients.

Pharmacologic Therapy

Guidelines for the Management of Hypertension

Any health care provider involved in the care of hypertensive patients should be familiar with pub-

Table 6-6.

General Guidelines for Prescribing Pharmacotherapy for Smoking Cessation*

Who should receive pharmacotherapy for smoking cessation?	All smokers trying to quit, except in the presence of special circumstances. Special consideration should be given before using pharmacotherapy with selected populations: those with medical contraindications, those smoking fewer than 10 cigarettes per day, pregnant and breast-feeding women, and adolescent smokers.
What are the first-line pharmacotherapies recommended?	All five of the FDA-approved pharmacotherapies for smoking cessation are recommended, including bupropion SR, nicotine gum, nicotine inhaler, nicotine nasal spray, and the nicotine patch.
What factors should a clinician consider when choosing among the five first-line pharmacotherapies?	Because of the lack of sufficient data to rank-order these five medications, choice of a specific first-line pharmacotherapy must be guided by factors such as clinician familiarity with the medications, contraindications for selected patients, patient preference, previous patient experience with a specific pharmacotherapy (positive or negative), and patient characteristics (e.g., history of depression, concerns about weight gain).
Are pharmacotherapeutic treatments appropriate for lighter smokers (e.g., 10–15 cigarettes per day)?	If pharmacotherapy is used with lighter smokers, clinicians should consider reducing the dose of first-line nicotine replacement therapy (NRT) pharmacotherapies. No adjustments are necessary when using bupropion SR.
What second-line pharmacotherapies are recommended?	Clonidine and nortriptyline
When should second-line agents be used for treating tobacco dependence?	Consider prescribing second-line agents for patients unable to use first-line medications because of contraindications or for patients for whom first-line medications are not helpful. Monitor patients for the known side effects of second-line agents.
Which pharmacotherapies should be considered with patients particularly concerned about weight gain?	Bupropion SR and nicotine replacement therapies, in particular nicotine gum, have been shown to delay, but not prevent, weight gain.
Are there pharmacotherapies that should be especially considered in patients with a history of depression?	Bupropion SR and nortriptyline appear to be effective with this population.
Should nicotine replacement therapies be avoided in patients with a history of cardiovascular disease?	No. The nicotine patch in particular is safe and has been shown not to cause adverse cardiovascular effects.
May tobacco-dependence pharmacotherapies be used long term (e.g., 6 months or more)?	Yes. This approach may be helpful with smokers who report persistent withdrawal symptoms during the course of pharmacotherapy or who desire long-term therapy. A minority of individuals who successfully quit smoking use ad libitum NRT medications (gum, nasal spray, inhaler) long term. The use of these medications long term does not present a known health risk. Additionally, the FDA has approved the use of bupropion SR for a long-term maintenance indication.
May pharmacotherapies ever be combined?	Yes. There is evidence that combining the nicotine patch with either nicotine gum or nicotine nasal spray increases long-term abstinence rates over those produced by a single form of NRT.

*Fiore MC, Bailey WC, Cohen SJ et al. Treating tobacco use and dependence. Quick reference guide for clinicians. Rockville, MD: U.S. Department of Health and Human Services. Public Health Service. October 2000. (No reprint permission necessary)

Table 6-7.
Suggestions for the Clinical Use of Pharmacotherapy for Smoking Cessation*

Pharmacotherapy	Precautions/ Contraindications	Side Effects	Dosage	Duration	Availability
Bupropion SR	History of seizure History of eating disorder	Insomnia Dry mouth	150 mg every morning for 3 days, then 150 mg twice daily (begin treatment 1–2 weeks prequit)	7–12 weeks maintenance up to 6 months	Zyban (prescription only)
Nicotine gum		Mouth soreness Dyspepsia	1–24 cigarettes per day = 2 mg of gum (up to 24 pieces per day) 25+ cigarettes per day = 4 mg of gum (up to 24 pieces per day)	Up to 12 weeks	Nicorette, Nicorette Mint (OTC only)
Nicotine inhaler		Local irritation of mouth and throat	6–16 cartridges/day	Up to 6 months	Nicotrol Inhaler (prescription only)
Nicotine nasal spray		Nasal irritation	8–40 doses/day	3–6 months	Nicotrol NS (prescription only)
Nicotine patch**		Local skin reaction Insomnia	21 mg/24 hours 14 mg/24 hours 7 mg/24 hours 15 mg/16 hours	4 weeks then 2 weeks then 2 weeks 8 weeks	Nicoderm CQ (OTC only), generic patches (prescription and OTC), Nicotrol (OTC only)
Clonidine	Rebound hypertension	Dry mouth Drowsiness Dizziness Sedation	0.15–0.75 mg/day	3–10 weeks	Oral generic clonidine, Catapres (prescription only) Transdermal Catapres (prescription only)
Nortriptyline	Risk of arrhythmias	Sedation Dry mouth	75–100 mg/day	12 weeks	Generic nortriptyline HCl (prescription only)

*The information contained within this table is not comprehensive. Please see package insert for additional information. OTC = over the counter; Fiore MC, Bailey WC, Cohen SJ et al. Treating tobacco use and dependence. Quick reference guide for clinicians. Rockville, MD: U.S. Department of Health and Human Services. Public Health Service. October 2000. (No reprint permission necessary)

**Generic brands of the patch recently became available and may be less expensive.

lished treatment guidelines on the management of hypertension. These guidelines serve as an invaluable tool in initiating, evaluating, and optimizing drug therapy regimens. Two sets of guidelines for the management of hypertensive patients are commonly used in clinical practice. They include the seventh report of the Joint National Committee on Prevention, Detection, Evaluation, and Treatment of High Blood Pressure[1] (JNC 7) and the 2003 European Society of Hypertension–European Society of Cardiology Guidelines for the Management of Arterial Hypertension (ESH–ESC).[60] Information from both sets of guidelines has been presented throughout this book. Although both publications are relatively similar in their recommendations for hypertensive drug therapy, the JNC 7 guidelines

Table 6-8.
Key Antihypertensive Trials*

Reference	Design; Patient Population	Drug and Dose	Outcomes	Comments
AASK[75]	R;1094 AA (18–70 years old) with renal insufficiency and HTN. Tx groups: MAP 102–107 mm Hg or MAP ≤92 mm Hg. Follow-up = 3–6.4 years.	Metoprolol 50–200 mg/d, or ramipril 2.5–10 mg/d, or amlodipine 5–10 mg/d.	Reduction of GFR by ≥50%, ESRD, or death: 22% ↓ with ramipril vs metoprolol (p=0.04), 38% ↓ with ramipril vs amlodipine (p=0.004).	Primary objective: To compare two different target BP goals and three antihypertensive agents on the progression of renal disease in hypertensive AA patients. Other agents could be added to achieve BP goals. Outcomes were secondary endpoint of the trial. There was no difference in the incidence of GFR reduction by ≥50%, ESRD, or death between those patients in the lower BP group than those patients in the higher BP group.
ABCD[76]	R, blinded; 470 patients (40–74 years old) with DM and DBP >80 mm Hg. Duration = 5 years.	Nisoldipine 10–60 mg/d vs enalapril 5–40 mg/d.	Fatal and nonfatal MI: 5 enalapril vs 25 nisoldipine (p=0.001). Nonfatal MI: 5 enalapril vs 22 nisoldipine (p=0.001).	Primary objective: To compare the effects of ACE I and CCB on CV outcomes in hypertensive patients with DM. Patients were divided into intensive treatment group with goal of decreasing DBP by 10 mm Hg or moderate treatment with no target decrease in DBP. Moderate treatment group could be randomized to receive placebo; open label antihypertensives could be used to control BP. CV outcomes were a secondary endpoint of the trial.
ALLHAT[61,77]	R, DB; 33,357 patients, >55 years old, stage 1 or 2 hypertension + ≥1 CV risk factor. Mean follow-up = 4.9 years.	Chlorthalidone 12.5–25 mg, or amlodipine 2.5–10 mg, or lisinopril 10–40 mg QD, or doxazosin 1–8 mg QD.	Fatal or nonfatal MI: chlorthalidone 0.3%, amlodipine 0.4%, lisinopril 0.4% (NS). Stroke: chlorthalidone 0.2%, lisinopril 0.3% (p=0.02). Heart failure: chlorthalidone 0.3% vs lisinopril 0.4% (p<0.001); chlorthalidone vs amlodipine 0.4% (p<0.001).	Primary objective: To compare the effects of ACE I, CCB, and alpha-blockers to chlorthalidone on CV events in hypertensive patients. Other agents (reserpine, clonidine, atenolol, and/or hydralazine) could be added to control BP. Doxazosin arm was discontinued prematurely due to lack of effectiveness in preventing CV events, particularly CHF; risk of CHF: doxazosin 8.13% vs chlorthalidone 4.45%, RR = 2.04 (95% CI 1.79–2.32, p< 0.001). Most patients required ≥ two drugs to control BP. Chlorthalidone is equally effective in preventing CV outcomes and less expensive than other agents.

(continued)

Table 6-8. *(continued)*
Key Antihypertensive Trials*

Reference	Design; Patient Population	Drug and Dose	Outcomes	Comments
ANBP 2[66]	R, OL; 6083 patients 65–84 years old with mean BP 168±13/91±8 mm Hg. Median follow-up = 4.1 years.	Enalapril or other ACE I, HCTZ, or other diuretic; doses not specified.	No difference in CV events or deaths from any cause between groups; 17% ↓ in all and first CV events in males treated with ACE I, HR 0.83 (95% CI 0.71–0.97).	Primary objective: To compare the effects of ACE I and diuretics on CV events in older hypertensive patients. Generally healthy and predominantly Caucasian patients with <10% CHD, CV disease, DM, or smoking. Choice of agent and dose made by individual family practitioner. 95% patients were Caucasian. Other agents could be added to control BP. More than half of the patients received monotherapy.
CAPPP[78]	R, OL;10,985 patients (25–66 years old) with DBP ≥100 mm Hg. Mean follow-up = 6.1 years.	Captopril 50–200 mg/d vs "conventional" treatment of diuretics, BB, or both.	No difference between groups in primary outcome of MI, stroke, and CV death, RR 1.05 (95% CI 0.9–1.22). Nonfatal and fatal stroke was higher in captopril group, RR 1.25 (95% CI 1.01–1.55).	Primary objective: To compare the effects of ACE I to diuretics, BB, or both on CV outcomes in hypertensive patients. Most commonly used BB: atenolol or metoprolol 50–100 mg/d; most commonly used diuretics: HCTZ 25 mg/d or bendroflumethiazide 2.5 mg/d. A diuretic could be added to captopril group; a CCB could be added to either group.
FACET[79]	R, OL; 380 patients with hypertension and DM. Follow-up = 3.5 years.	Fosinopril 20 mg/day or amlodipine 10 mg/day.	Patients treated with fosinopril had a lower risk of MI, stroke, or hospitalized angina vs patients treated with amlodipine, HR 0.47 (95% CI 0.26–0.95).	Primary objective: To compare the effects of ACE I and CCB on lipids and DM in patients with hypertension and DM. If BP was not controlled on one drug, the other study drug could be added. CV outcomes were a secondary endpoint of the trial.
HOT[80]	R; 18,790 patients (mean age 61.5± 7.5 SD) with DBP 100–115 mm Hg assigned to target DBP groups: ≤90 mm Hg, ≤85 mm Hg, ≤80 mm Hg. Average follow-up = 3.8 years.	Felodipine 5–10 mg/d; additional therapy included ACE I or BB, diuretic.	In patients with DM, 51% reduction in major CV events in patients with DBP ≤80 mm Hg vs patients with DBP ≤90 mm Hg.	Primary objective: To assess the optimal target diastolic BP and the benefit of low-dose aspirin in hypertensive patients.

(continued)

Table 6-8. *(continued)*
Key Antihypertensive Trials*

Reference	Design; Patient Population	Drug and Dose	Outcomes	Comments
INSIGHT[81]	R, DB; 6321 patients 55–80 years old with BP >150/95 mm Hg or SBP ≥160 mm Hg + ≥1 CV risk factor.	Nifedipine LA GITS 30–60 mg/day vs HCTZ 25–50 mg/amiloride 2.5–5 mg/d; atenolol 25–50 mg or enalapril 5–10 mg/d could be added.	Combined CV outcomes: 6.3% nifedipine vs 5.8% diuretic group, RR 1.1 (95% CI 0.91–1.34). Fatal MI: 0.5% nifedipine vs 0.2% diuretic, RR 3.22 (95% CI 1.18–8.80). Non-fatal CHF: 0.8% nifedipine vs 0.3% diuretic, RR 2.2 (95% CI 1.07–4.49).	Primary objective: To compare the effects of CCB and diuretic on CV outcomes in hypertensive patients with CV risk factors. No difference in combined outcome of CV mortality, MI, CHF, or stroke between two groups. Less fatal MI and CHF with diuretic group; more dropouts in nifedipine group due to peripheral edema (p<0.0001).
LIFE[62]	R, DB; 9193 patients with stage 1 or 2 hypertension and LVH. Mean follow-up = 4.8 years.	Atenolol 50–100 mg QD; losartan 50–100 mg QD.	CV mortality, stroke, and MI: losartan 11%, atenolol 13% (p=0.021); stroke: losartan 5%, atenolol 7% (p=0.001); new-onset diabetes: losartan 6%, atenolol 8% (p=0.001).	Primary objective: To compare the effects of losartan and atenolol on CV outcomes in hypertensive patients with LVH. HCTZ and other BP meds could be added to control BP; most patients required ≥2 drugs to control BP.
MIDAS[82]	R, DB; 883 patients (mean age = 58.5±8.5 years) with diastolic HTN. Follow-up = 3 years.	Isradipine 2.5–5 mg BID vs HCTZ 12.5–25 mg BID; enalapril 2.5–10 mg BID could be added to control BP.	Higher incidence of angina (RR 3.66, 95% CI 1.03–13.2) and vascular events/procedures (RR 1.63, 95% CI 1.08–2.47).	Primary objective of the study was to determine the rate of progression of intimal medial thickness between patients receiving isradipine and HCTZ.
NORDIL[63]	R, OL; 10,881 patients (50–74 years old) with DBP ≥100 mm Hg. Mean follow-up = 4.5 years.	Diltiazem 180–360 mg/d vs thiazide diuretic, BB, or both.	No difference between groups in the incidence of stroke, MI, or CV death, RR 1.00 (95% CI 0.87–1.15). Lower incidence of stroke in diltiazem group, RR 0.8 (95% CI 0.65–0.99).	Primary objective: To compare the effects of CCB to diuretics, BB, or both on CV outcomes in hypertensive patients. Other agents could be added (ACE I, diuretics, BB, and others) to control BP.
SHEP[64]	R, DB, PC; 4736 patients ≥60 years old with SBP 160–219 mm Hg and DBP <90 mm Hg. Follow-up = 5 years.	Chlorthalidone 12.5–25 mg/d; could be changed to atenolol 25–50 mg/d or reserpine 0.05–1 mg/d if needed.	Incidence of stroke: 5.2% treatment group vs 8.2% placebo, RR = 0.64 (p=0.0003).	Primary objective: To evaluate the effect of drug treatment on the incidence of stroke in patients with ISH.

(continued)

Table 6-8. *(continued)*
Key Antihypertensive Trials*

Reference	Design; Patient Population	Drug and Dose	Outcomes	Comments
STOP-2[65]	R, OL; 6614 patients 70–84 years old with SBP >180, DBP >105 mm Hg, or both. Follow-up = 5 years.	Conventional group (atenolol 50 mg/d, metoprolol 100 mg/d, pindolol 5 mg/d, or HCTZ 25 mg + amiloride 2.5 mg/d) vs newer group ACE I (enalapril 10 mg/d or lisinopril 10 mg/d); or CCB (felodipine 2.5 mg/d or isradipine 2.5 mg/d).	NS difference in combined endpoint of fatal stroke or CV disease between conventional and newer therapies, RR = 0.99 (95% CI 0.84–1.16).	Primary objective: To compare the effects of "conventional" therapy to "newer" therapies on CV outcomes in older hypertensive patients. Mean supine BP at baseline: 194/98 mm Hg; no difference in BP lowering between groups. Patients were randomized to conventional or newer therapies, but no randomization occurred between groups. More than 1/3 of patients were not receiving their randomized treatment at the end of the trial.
Syst-Eur[67]	R, DB, PC; 4695 patients ≥60 years old with SBP 160–219 mm Hg and DBP <95 mm Hg. Mean follow-up = 2 years.	Nitrendipine 10–40 mg/d ± enalapril 5–20 mg/d ± HCTZ 12.5–25 mg/d vs placebo.	Patients with DM, treatment vs placebo: 70% ↓ in CV mortality (p=0.01), 62% ↓ in CV events (p=0.002), and 69% ↓ in stroke (p=0.02). Patients without DM, treatment vs placebo: 25% ↓ in CV events (p=0.02), 36% ↓ in stroke (p=0.02).	Primary objective: To compare the effects of CCB to placebo in hypertensive patients with and without DM. Enalapril and HCTZ could be added or substituted for nitrendipine to reach BP goal; 55% of the treatment group received nitrendipine only, 26% received nitrendipine + enalapril, 16% received nitrendipine + enalapril + HCTZ.
Syst-China[72]	R, DB, PC; 2394 patients ≥60 years old with SBP 160–219 mm Hg; Median follow-up = 3 years.	Nitrendipine 10–40 mg/day ± captopril 12.5–50 mg/day ± HCTZ 12.5–50 mg/d vs placebo.	All cause mortality: 39% ↓ in treatment group (p=0.0003); stroke: 58% ↓ in treatment group (p=0.02); CV mortality: 39% ↓ in treatment group (p=0.03).	Primary objective: To compare the effects of treatment to placebo on stroke and CV complications. Study participants were Chinese. 73.5% of treatment group received nitrendipine monotherapy, 20.4% received captopril, 3% received HCTZ, and 3.1% received other antihypertensive drugs.

*AA = African-Americans; ACE I= angiotensin-converting-enzyme inhibitor; BB = beta-blockers, BP = blood pressure; CCB = calcium channel blockers; CHD = coronary heart disease; CI = confidence interval; CHF = congestive heart failure; CV = cardiovascular; d = day; DB = double-blind; DBP = diastolic blood pressure, DM = diabetes mellitus; ESRD = end-stage renal disease; GITS = gastrointestinal transport system; GFR = glomerular filtration rate; HCTZ = hydrochlorothiazide; HR = hazard ratio; HTN = hypertension; ISH = isolated systolic hypertension; LA = long-acting; LVH = left ventricular hypertrophy; MAP = mean arterial pressure; MI = myocardial infarction; NS = not significant; OL = open-label; PC = placebo-controlled; R = randomized; RR = relative risk; SBP = systolic blood pressure, SD = standard deviation; Tx = treatment; vs = versus.

strive to base all recommendations on evidence-based literature. For this reason, the JNC 7 guidelines are reviewed here in more detail than the ESH–ESC guidelines.

The JNC 7 guidelines recommend a thiazide-type diuretic (e.g., hydrochlorothiazide) either alone or in combination with other agents for ini-tial treatment of hypertension in most patients. This is due to data supporting improvement in morbidity and mortality in patients with hypertension and the number of outcomes trials using thiazide-type diuretics in combination with other agents.[1,61–65] In addition, diuretics are available in generic formulation and are inexpensive. Several

Table 6-9.
Combination Agents for the Treatment of Hypertension[1]

Combination Type*	Fixed-Dose Combination, mg**	Trade Name
ACEIs and CCBs	Amlodipine/benazepril hydrochloride (2.5/10, 5/10, 5/20, 10/20)	Lotrel
	Enalapril maleate/felodipine (5/5)	Lexxel
	Trandolapril/verapamil (2/180, 1/240, 2/240, 4/240)	Tarka
ACEIs and diuretics	Benazepril/hydrochlorothiazide (5/6.25, 10/12.5, 20/12.5, 20/25)	Lotensin HCT
	Captopril/hydrochlorothiazide (25/15, 25/25, 50/l5, 50/25)	Capozide
	Enalapril maleate/hydrochlorothiazide (5/12.5, 10/25)	Vaseretic
	Lisinopril/hydrochlorothiazide (10/12.5, 20/12.5, 20/25)	Prinzide
	Moexipril HCI/hydrochlorothiazide (7.5/12.5, l5/25)	Uniretic
	Quinapril HCI/hydrochiorothiazide (10/12.5, 20/12.5, 20/25)	Accuretic
ARBs and diuretics	Candesartan cilexetil/hydrochlorothiazide (16/12.5, 32/12.5)	Atacand HCT
	Eprosartan mesylate/hydrochlorothiazide (600/12.5, 600/25)	Teveten/HCT
	Irbesartan/hydrochlorothiazide (l50/12.5, 300/12.5)	Avalide
	Iosartan potassium/hydrochlorothiazide (50/12.5, 100/25)	Hyzaar
	Telmisartan/hydrochlorothiazide (40/12.5, 80/12.5)	Micardis/HCT
	Valsartan/hydrochlorothiazide (80/12.5, 160/12.5)	Diovan/HCT
BBs and diuretics	Atenolol/chlorthalidone (50/25, 100/25)	Tenoretic
	Bisoprolol fumarate/hydrochlorothiazide (2.5/6.25, 5/6.25, 10/6.25)	Ziac
	Propranolol LA/hydrochlorothiazide (40/25, 80/25)	Inderide
	Metoprolol tartrate/hydrochlorothiazide (50/25, 100/25)	Lopressor HCT
	Nadolol/bendroflumethiazide (40/5, 80/5)	Corzide
	Timolol maleate/hydrochlorothiazide (10/25)	Timolide
Centrally acting drug and diuretic	Methyldopa/hydrochlorothiazide (250/15, 250/25, 500/30, 500/50)	Aldoril
	Reserpine/chlorothiazide (0.125/250, 0.25/500)	Diupres
	Reserpine/hydrochlorothiazide (0.125/25, 0.125/50)	Hydropres
Diuretic and diuretic	Amiloride HCI/hydrochlorothiazide (5/50)	Moduretic
	Spironolactone/hydrochlorothiazide (25/25, 50/50)	Aldactone
	Triamterene/hydrochlorothiazide (37.5/25, 50/25, 75/50)	Dyazide, Maxzide

*Drug abbreviations: ACEI, angiotensin converting enzyme inhibitor; ARB, angiotensin receptor blocker; BB, beta-blocker; CCB, calcium channel blocker.

**Some drug combinations are available in multiple fixed doses. Each drug dose is reported in milligrams.

Adapted from the seventh report of the Joint National Committee on Prevention, Detection, Evaluation, and Treatment of High Blood Pressure. National Heart, Lung, and Blood Institute, National Institutes of Health, May 2003; NIH publication no. 03-5233.

other classes of antihypertensive agents, including angiotensin-converting-enzyme (ACE) inhibitors, angiotensin receptor blockers (ARBs), beta-blockers (BBs), and calcium channel blockers (CCBs), have demonstrated benefit on cardiovascular and/or cerebrovascular disease in well-designed outcomes trials and may be recommended as first-line treatment in certain patients.[61–63,66,67] For more details on the results of these and other antihypertensive trials, see **Table 6-8** in which several key trials are summarized.

Several clinical trials have found that many patients require two or more antihypertensive agents to control blood pressure.[1,61,62,67] When a second antihypertensive agent is indicated, JNC 7 recommends the addition of a drug from a different class.[1] In many cases, diuretics may make other antihypertensive therapies more effective and should be considered as add-on therapy if not chosen as the initial agent.[1] When the systolic blood pressure (SBP) or diastolic blood pressure (DBP) is greater than 20 and 10 mm Hg above the target, respectively (i.e., patients with stage 2 hypertension), consideration may be given to initiating therapy with two agents at the same time.[1] (**Table 6-9** lists several combination antihypertensive agents.) However, certain patients, such as the elderly, those with diabetes, or those with autonomic dysfunction, may be at risk for developing orthostatic hypotension and should be monitored closely.[1]

Patients presenting with significantly elevated blood pressure, or stage 2 hypertension, should be evaluated for signs and symptoms of immediate organ damage.[1] JNC 7 defines this as acute target organ damage and includes such conditions as encephalopathy, myocardial infarction, unstable angina, pulmonary edema, eclampsia, stroke, head trauma, life-threatening arterial bleeding, and aortic dissection.[1] When both factors are present, hospitalization and injectable antihypertensive treatments are usually required. If patients present with elevated blood pressure or stage 2 hypertension without the presence of immediate organ damage, JNC 7 recommends evaluation, close monitoring, and the administration of combination oral antihypertensive agents.[1] In previous JNC guidelines, terms such as hypertensive urgency and emergency generally referred to patients with SBP greater than 180 mm Hg and DBP greater than 110 mm Hg (stage 3 or 4 hypertension). More recent JNC guidelines consolidated the classification of blood pressure into stage 1 and 2 hypertension and focused more on the presence of clinical signs and symptoms to guide management.[1]

Concomitant Disease States That Influence Antihypertensive Therapy

Certain concomitant medical conditions affect antihypertensive therapy decisions. Several antihypertensive agents have been shown to improve morbidity and/or mortality when used to treat other diseases. Examples include the use of BBs to prevent reinfarction and mortality in patients who have a history of myocardial infarction or the use of an ARB or ACE inhibitor to slow progression and de-

lay the onset of nephropathy in patients with diabetes. When appropriate, the choice of antihypertensive agent should also treat a coexisting disease.

JNC 7 recommends the choice of initial antihypertensive therapy be based on the presence or absence of compelling indications.[1] These indications include heart failure, postmyocardial infarction, high risk for coronary artery disease, diabetes, chronic kidney disease, and recurrent stroke prevention. In patients with a compelling indication, drug therapy should be focused on those agents with proven beneficial effects. Due to the risk of hypertension in patients with prehypertension (SBP 120–139 mm Hg or DBP 80–89 mm Hg) and the benefit of specific agents in certain disease states, drug therapy is recommended in patients with prehypertension and a compelling indication.[1] If no such indications are present, JNC 7 recommends including thiazide diuretics in the initial treatment of hypertension. JNC 7 recommendations for drug therapy in patients with various disease states can be found in **Table 6-10**. Considerations for antihypertensive therapy in patients with select indications can be found in **Table 6-11**.

Conversely, some antihypertensive agents have unfavorable effects on concomitant diseases and should be avoided when possible. Examples in which certain disease states limit the use of specific drugs include the use of BBs in patients with reactive airway disease or the use of reserpine in patients with depression. **Table 6-12** lists several precautions to specific antihypertensive agents.

Effectiveness of Antihypertensive Therapy in Select Populations

One factor that may affect hypertensive drug therapy decisions is age, both young and old. Compared to elderly patients, hypertension in children and adolescents is relatively uncommon although the incidence is increasing. Once secondary causes have been ruled out, the treatment of hypertension in children and adolescents is similar to that of adults. However, drug therapy should only be employed if lifestyle modification is clearly inadequate. For a more detailed review of hypertension in this population, the National High Blood Pressure Education Program published an updated report in 1996.[68]

As discussed in Chapter 1 SBP continues to rise as a person ages, while DBP reaches a plateau and may even decrease. Elderly patients commonly have isolated systolic hypertension (ISH), defined as a

Table 6-10.
JNC 7 Recommendations for Use of Antihypertensive Agents in Concomitant Disease States*

Disease State	Recommended Drug Therapy	Comments
Acute coronary syndrome (ACS)	BB + ACE I	BBs are beneficial in ACS due to decrease myocardial workload and oxygen demands. ACE Is are also recommended in the ACC/AHA guidelines for ACS patients with hypertension.[83,84]
Angina pectoris, stable	BB or CCB	BB and CCB reduce myocardial oxygen demand and are useful in treating hypertensive patients with angina. BBs are preferred initial therapy in patients with stable angina.[85] Short-acting calcium channel blockers (e.g., immediate-release nifedipine) should be avoided in patients with hypertension.[74]
Diabetes mellitus**	ACE I- or ARB-based regimen	ACE Is have been shown to slow the progression and delay the initiation of nephropathy in patients with diabetes.[86] They have also been found to slow the progression of nephropathy in patients with type 2 diabetes mellitus with or without hypertension[87–89] and data suggest ACE Is are beneficial in diabetic patients without proteinuria.[90] Irbesartan has been shown to decrease the progression of nephropathy in patients with type 2 diabetes mellitus, hypertension, and evidence of nephropathy (proteinuria plus elevated serum creatinine).[91] Two or more drugs are often needed to control BP in patients with DM.[92,93]
	Thiazide diuretics, BB, and CCB are also beneficial.	Thiazide diuretics, BB, ACE I, ARB, and CCB have been found to decrease CV disease and stroke in patients with DM.[61,62]
Heart failure, asymptomatic LV dysfunction	ACE I + BB	ACE Is should be used in all patients with a low left ventricular ejection fraction as they have been shown to improve survival and reduce morbidity in patients with heart failure.[94] Carvedilol, bisoprolol, and metoprolol XL have all been shown to reduce morbidity and mortality in patients with mild-to-moderate heart failure.[95–98]
Heart failure, symptomatic or end-stage LV dysfunction**	ACE I, BB, ARB, aldosterone antagonist, loop diuretic	ACE I, BB, ARB, aldosterone antagonists and loop diuretics have all been shown to be beneficial in the treatment of patients with heart failure.[99–101]
Myocardial infarction, status post	BB, ACE I, aldosterone antagonist	BBs have been shown to reduce mortality and reinfarction in patients who have had an MI.[102] BB with intrinsic sympathomimetic activity (ISA), including acebutolol, carteolol, pindolol, and penbutolol, should be avoided in this population. ACE Is have been shown to reduce mortality and the development of heart failure in certain high-risk patients following an MI.[102] As add-on therapy, eplerenone has been shown to decrease morbidity and mortality in post-MI patients with left ventricular dysfunction.[103]
High coronary disease risk**	Diuretic, BB, ACE I, CCB	Several trials in patients with high risk for coronary artery disease found beneficial effects in CV morbidity and mortality when diuretics, BB, ACE I, or CCB were used.[61,62,66,90,104]
Chronic kidney disease**	ACE I or ARB	ACE I and ARB may slow the progression of renal disease in patients with or without DM.[75,91,105,106] A loop diuretic may be needed in combination with other antihypertensive agents in patients with a GFR <30 ml/min.
Stroke, recurrent**	ACE I + thiazide diuretic	Combination therapy with ACE I + thiazide diuretic has been shown to reduce the risk of recurrent stroke.[107]

*ACC = American College of Cardiology; ACE I = angiotensin-converting-enzyme inhibitor; AHA = American Heart Association; ARB = angiotensin receptor blocker; BB = beta-blocker; BP = blood pressure; CCB = calcium channel blocker; DM = diabetes mellitus; LV = left ventricular; and MI = myocardial infarction.

**Denotes compelling indications per JNC 7 guidelines.

Table 6-11.

Beneficial Effects of Antihypertensive Therapies in Select Indications*

Disease State	Drug Therapy	Comments
Atrial fibrillation	BB, CCB	BB and nondihydropyridine CCB are useful for ventricular rate control in patients with atrial fibrillation.
Cyclosporine-induced hypertension	CCB	Diltiazem and verapamil can increase serum cyclosporine concentrations, while nifedipine and isradipine have little to no effect.[108]
Essential tremor	BB	Noncardioselective BB, such as propranolol, are preferred.
Osteoporosis	Thiazide diuretics	Thiazide diuretics may be useful in patients with osteoporosis because they decrease renal calcium excretion.
Preoperative hypertension	BB	Atenolol has been shown to reduce perioperative cardiac morbidity and mortality in patients with or at risk for cardiovascular disease.[109]
Benign prostatic hypertrophy (BPH)	Alpha blockers	Alpha adrenergic blockers have been shown to increase urinary flow and improve symptoms of BPH, including frequency of urination, nocturia, urgency, and incontinence. Although these agents relieve symptoms of BPH, they are not as effective as diuretics in reducing cardiovascular endpoints in patients with hypertension and should not be used as first-line agents in hypertensive patients with BPH.[77]

*Adapted from the seventh report of the Joint National Committee on Prevention, Detection, Evaluation, and Treatment of High Blood Pressure. National Heart, Lung, and Blood Institute, National Institutes of Health, May 2003; NIH publication no. 03-5233.

SBP higher than 140 mm Hg and a DBP less than 90 mm Hg. In this population, SBP tends to be a more important determinant of target organ damage (TOD) (e.g., cardiovascular and cerebrovascular diseases, heart failure, and renal failure) and death.[69] The target blood pressure is still less than 140/90 mm Hg for patients with ISH. However for some patients with a very elevated SBP (e.g., 180 mm Hg or more), it may be reasonable to achieve the target blood pressure at a much slower pace and attempt a temporary target SBP of 160 mm Hg.[1] Further complicating matters is that elderly patients may have pseudohypertension (discussed in detail in Chapter 3), resulting in falsely elevated blood pressure readings. Pseudohypertension may be suspected in patients with elevated blood pressure in the absence of TOD.

Several clinical trials evaluating antihypertensive therapies in the elderly have demonstrated significant reductions in stroke and/or cardiovascular disease.[64,67,70–72] Due to the overwhelming benefit of thiazide diuretics in reducing stroke, heart failure,

and myocardial infarction, these agents are recommended for initial treatment of elderly patients with hypertension.[1,64,70,71] BBs may be combined with thiazide diuretics if blood pressure cannot be controlled with one agent alone.[1,64] In fact, many of the patients in the clinical trials were receiving a combination of a BB and a thiazide diuretic. Evidence is emerging that long-acting dihydropyridine calcium channel antagonists are also beneficial in reducing strokes in elderly patients with ISH and represent a reasonable alternative for elderly patients who are unable to tolerate thiazide diuretics or need additional blood pressure control.[1,67,72]

Elderly patients can be more sensitive to the effects of medications, particularly volume depletion and sympathetic activation. Frail, elderly patients tend to have the most difficulty with medications and antihypertensive therapy should be initiated at the lowest possible dose in these patients. For example, hydrochlorothiazide should be initiated at 12.5 mg per day. Blood pressure should be monitored closely, particularly for the presence of ortho-

Table 6-12.
Antihypertensive Therapy Precautions in Select Indications*

Disease State	Drug Therapy	Precaution
Asthma/chronic obstructive pulmonary disease	BB	BB may cause bronchospasm due to the blockade of beta receptors in the lungs. BB should be used cautiously in patients with reactive airway disease. If indicated, β_1 selective or cardioselective agents (i.e., acebutolol, atenolol, betaxolol, bisoprolol, or metoprolol) should be considered and patients should be monitored for symptoms of bronchospasm.
Depression	BB, centrally acting alpha agonists, reserpine	BB may worsen depression and should be used cautiously in this population. Depression has been reported in up to 30% of hypertensive patients receiving reserpine. Because centrally acting alpha agonists and reserpine have been associated with depression, these agents should be avoided if possible.
Angioedema	ACE I	ACE I should be avoided in patients with angioedema.
Gout	Diuretics	Diuretics may increase serum uric acid levels and cause gouty flares in patients with a history of gout. Additionally, increases in uric acid may contribute adversely to cardiovascular events.[110] ACE I and angiotensin II receptor antagonists may blunt diuretic-induced increases in uric acid.
Hyponatremia	Thiazide diuretics	Thiazide diuretics should be used with caution in patients with history of hyponatremia.
2nd or 3rd degree heart block	BB, CCB	BB and CCB should be avoided in patients with preexisting heart block due to their actions in lowering heart rate.
Liver disease	Labetalol, methyldopa	Labetalol and methyldopa have been associated with significant hepatic injury and should be avoided in patients with liver disease.
Pregnancy	ACE I, angiotensin II receptor blockers	ACE I and angiotensin II receptor blockers are teratogenic and should be avoided in hypertensive pregnant women.[111]
Renal insufficiency	Potassium-sparing diuretics	Potassium-sparing agents, such as spironolactone or amiloride, may aggravate hyperkalemia in patients with renal insufficiency.
Renovascular disease	ACE I, ARB	ACE I and angiotensin II receptor blockers may cause acute renal failure in patients with renal artery stenosis.

*Adapted from the seventh report of the Joint National Committee on Prevention, Detection, Evaluation, and Treatment of High Blood Pressure. National Heart, Lung, and Blood Institute, National Institutes of Health, May 2003; NIH publication no. 03-5233.

static hypotension, and the medication should be titrated slowly.

Although young males may have a higher incidence of hypertension than females, gender generally does not change the course of disease progression or outcome. Currently, there is no evidence to support different treatment approaches for hypertensive men and women based on gender alone.[73] Women developing hypertension as a result of oral contraceptive use should consider alternative meth-ods or medications for contraception.[1] Hypertensive women who are or plan to become pregnant should avoid the use of ACE inhibitors and ARBs. A list of antihypertensive therapies used to treat these patients can be found in **Table 6-13**.

The prevalence of hypertension in the United States varies by race. African-Americans, in particular, have a higher incidence of hypertension and poorer outcomes related to the disease.[1] This is thought to be due, in part, to delay in the initiation

Table 6-13.
Antihypertensive Drugs Used in Pregnancy*

The report of the NHBPEP Working Group on High Blood Pressure in Pregnancy permits continuation of drug therapy in women with chronic hypertension (except for ACE inhibitors). In addition, angiotensin II receptor blockers should not be used during pregnancy. In women with chronic hypertension with diastolic levels of 100 mm Hg or greater (lower when end organ damage or underlying renal disease is present) and in women with acute hypertension when levels are 105 mm Hg or greater, the following agents are suggested.

Suggested	Drug Comments
Central alpha-agonists	Methyldopa (C) is the drug of choice recommended by the NHBPEP Working Group.
Beta-blockers	Atenolol (C) and metoprolol (C) appear to be safe and effective in late pregnancy. Labetalol (C) also appears to be effective (alpha- and beta-blocker).
Calcium antagonists	Potential synergism with magnesium sulfate may lead to precipitous hypotension. (C)
ACE inhibitors, angiotensin II receptor blockers	Fetal abnormalities, including death, can be caused, and these drugs should not be used in pregnancy. (D)
Diuretics	Diuretics (C) are recommended for chronic hypertension if prescribed before gestation or if patients appear to be salt-sensitive. They are not recommended in preeclampsia.
Direct vasodilators	Hydralazine (C) is the parenteral drug of choice based on its long history of safety and efficacy. (C)

There are several other antihypertensive drugs for which there are very limited data. The U.S. Food and Drug Administration classifies pregnancy risk as follows: C, adverse effects in animals; no controlled trials in humans; use if risk appears justified; D, positive evidence of fetal risk. ACE indicates angiotensin-converting enzyme.

*Adapted from the sixth report of the Joint National Committee on Prevention, Detection, Evaluation, and Treatment of High Blood Pressure. National Heart, Lung, and Blood Institute, National Institutes of Health, November 1997; NIH publication no. 98-4080.

of treatment.[74] Modification of cardiovascular risk factors such as smoking cessation, obesity, and diabetes become especially important. Additionally, blood pressure in this group is sodium dependent and responds well to a reduction in dietary sodium.[74]

In general, the treatment of hypertension in the African-American population is consistent with other groups.[1] Hypertension in African-Americans differs from others in that blood pressure is more fluid and sodium dependent and plasma renin activity is reduced. Historically, thiazide diuretics and CCBs were commonly used as initial treatment due to their antihypertensive effects in this population. Other antihypertensive agents, ACE inhibitors, ARBs, and BBs, were commonly not used as monotherapy as blood pressure was not as responsive in this population. However, a recent large randomized trial evaluated the effects of BBs, CCBs, and ACE inhibitors in African-American individu-

als with hypertension and renal insufficiency and found that ACE inhibitors were more effective than BBs and CCBs in slowing the progression of renal disease in these patients.[75] Thiazide diuretics should still be considered as first-line therapy in hypertensive African-American patients without chronic kidney disease or other compelling indications and also as add-on therapy for all appropriate patients.[1]

Patient Considerations for Antihypertensive Therapy

After evaluating antihypertensive drug therapy for appropriateness in specific populations and concomitant disease states, consideration should be given to a number of patient-related factors before initiating drug therapy. Certain patient-related factors, such as age, sex, race, and concomitant medical conditions, may dictate which medications will provide the most benefit in the treatment of hypertension. After these factors are taken into consideration, other patient-related concerns should be addressed as well, such as medication expense, insurance coverage, previous adverse effect(s) to particular medication, and difficulty in adhering to the medication regimen.

Medication expense is an important consideration in determining antihypertensive drug therapy in patients with no prescription insurance or those with limited income. If the medication is expensive or represents a significant amount of the patient's monthly income, chances of nonadherence to therapy and subsequent adverse outcomes are great. Most classes of antihypertensive agents recommended as first-line therapy (i.e., BBs, ACE inhibitors, and thiazide diuretics) for hypertensive patients with and without compelling indications have generic agents available which are much less expensive. Appendix 6-2 lists websites that help indigent patients find assistance.

In instances where a proprietary medication is needed, qualifying patients may be able to obtain their medication at no charge from the manufacturer. In most cases, a request made to the manufacturer must be initiated through a health care provider. This process can be time consuming but well worth the effort if complications of untreated hypertension can be prevented.

Medication coverage, or the payment of medications through a third-party insurer or a state or federal assistance program, may also be a determinant for medication expense. It is becoming increasingly common for programs to utilize a formulary or "preferred" medication list. In most instances, a generic medication is preferred. Additionally, there usually are no restrictions on the class of antihypertensive agent used (e.g., ACE inhibitor or ARB) but certain proprietary products within a class may be restricted. Initiating therapy with an agent on the "restricted" list or one that is nonformulary usually results in a financial penalty to the patient (e.g., patient must pay a higher copay or purchase the medication out of pocket). Due to the number of different third-party payers that may insure patients in a particular area, keeping up with the "preferred" agents or memorizing a formulary can be quite a daunting task. In some areas, state professional societies or available computer programs may keep this information for the most common insurers.

The occurrence of adverse drug reactions may also guide the antihypertensive drug therapy regimen. Ideally, agents should be used that produce minimal adverse effects. Some adverse effects can be hazardous (e.g., development of acute renal failure in a patient receiving an ACE inhibitor), while others are annoying (e.g., development of a dry, hacking cough in a patient receiving an ACE inhibitor). The presence of annoying adverse effects may lead to nonadherence to therapy. In general, the offending agent should be discontinued and another agent from a different class should be initiated. An exception may occur when the offending agent is extremely beneficial to the patient. An example might be the presence of fatigue in a patient receiving BB therapy and who has had a myocardial infarction. The BB has been shown to improve mortality and decrease the chance of experiencing a subsequent myocardial infarction. However, the patient's quality of life is compromised. In these cases, the patient and health care provider should discuss the risks and benefits of therapy. The ultimate decision lies in the hands of the patient.

If adherence to the antihypertensive regimen is difficult, efforts should be made to simplify the regimen. Certainly with the number of antihypertensive agents available today, medications administered on a once-daily basis are preferred. Fortunately, the majority of antihypertensive agents can be given once or twice daily. The health care provider must also consider whether cost plays a role in nonadherence to therapy. If suspected, generic agents administered once daily are preferred (e.g., hydrochlorothiazide or atenolol).

Key Points for Patients

A patient should make the following lifestyle modifications to help control blood pressure:

Maintain weight at a Body Mass Index of 19–25.

- The BMI can be calculated as (weight in pounds $\times$ 703)/height in inches^2.

Increase physical activity.

- A patient should, at a minimum, walk briskly for at least 30 minutes on most days of the week.
- If a patient has a heart condition, he or she should consult with his or her physician about what level of exercise is safe.

Eat a healthy diet.

- Increase fresh fruits and vegetables and low-fat dairy products. Reduce content of total and saturated fat in diet.
- Avoid processed foods and do not use a saltshaker at the table; limit salty snacks.

Limit alcohol use.

- Alcohol consumption can lead to liver cirrhosis, cancer, and other causes of death. If a patient does consume alcohol, it should be kept to a minimum.
- Men should limit alcohol to 1 ounce a day (24 oz beer, 10 oz wine, 2 oz whisky).
- Women or men of slight build should limit alcohol to half an ounce per day (12 oz beer, 5 oz wine, 1 oz whisky).

Stop smoking or using other tobacco products.

- Remember it is never too late to quit.
- If a patient has tried and failed to quit before, remember that it takes many people several tries before they are successful.

Take antihypertensive medication(s) as prescribed.

- The use of antihypertensive drugs is very important to lower your blood pressure and prevent complications related to hypertension, such as having a heart attack or stroke, developing kidney failure, and blindness.
- Lowering blood pressure may help to improve quality of life by decreasing the risk of stroke or heart attack.
- If a patient has difficulty paying for medications, a less expensive alternative may be available or a program may assist with the medications.

Patient Cases

1 JS is a 52-year-old African-American male who presents with a blood pressure of 160/95 on repeated measurements. He has not had regular follow-up with a physician and has not received any treatment in the past for hypertension. His weight is 102 kg (224 pounds) and his height is 175 cm (69 inches). He smokes one pack of cigarettes per day, and he eats out frequently at fast food restaurants. He consumes three to five drinks per day on most weekends, but none during the week. He does not take any prescription medications, but he does take over-the-counter allergy medications (loratidine 10 mg QD; pseudoephedrine prn). His physician decides appropriately that drug therapy or even dual therapy is indicated. Since drug therapy will be started, JS is less than excited about the prospect at having to also implement lifestyle modification. What changes in lifestyle would JS benefit from?

JS is above his ideal body weight (BMI = 33) and is most likely on a higher salt and higher fat diet than recommended since he frequently eats convenience foods. He should receive individualized counseling on dietary modification to address weight loss and sodium and fat reduction. His smoking history is another major risk factor predisposing him for atherosclerotic heart disease, and he should be counseled on the benefits of smoking cessation. His alcohol intake could be viewed as binge drinking, which may cause acute rises in blood pressure. In addition, the alcohol intake at these amounts is a significant caloric source in his diet. He should be counseled to reduce intake to one or two drinks at one time. His nonprescription drug intake should be addressed. He should avoid systemic decongestants, since his blood pressure is uncontrolled. JS should be questioned about his progress in making lifestyle changes at each encounter, since education has been shown to provide additional lowering of blood pressure.

2 EM is a 62-year-old African-American male with newly diagnosed hypertension. His past medical history includes depression and occasional gastroesophageal reflux disease. His blood pressure (BP) today is 145/80 mm Hg, which is consistent with several other office and home BP measurements. He has been successful in lowering his systolic BP by 5 mm Hg through lifestyle modification. However, it is still elevated. His current medications include sertraline 50 mg QD and Mylanta® prn. Baseline labs, including potassium, serum creatinine, urinalysis, complete blood count, fasting glucose, and fasting lipid profile, were all within normal limits. In addition, no abnormalities were found on the ECG. Which antihypertensive therapy would you recommend for EM?

Hydrochlorothiazide 12.5 mg QD would be a good initial choice for EM. JNC 7 guidelines recommend initial antihypertensive therapy with a thiazide diuretic in the absence of other compelling indications due to evidence supporting an improvement in mortality and the low cost. Although BBs, ACE inhibitors, and ARBs may not be as effective in lowering blood pressure in this population when used alone, combination therapy with a diuretic has produced favorable effects on blood pressure and should be considered when and if another drug is needed to adequately control blood pressure.

3 DL is a 53-year-old Caucasian male with a history of hypertension, coronary artery disease, osteoarthritis of the knees, and dyslipidemia. He is adherent with his lifestyle modifications. His current medications include hydrochlorothiazide 25 mg QD, aspirin 81 mg QD, simvastatin 20 mg QD, acetaminophen 500 mg two tablets QID, and sublingual nitroglycerin 0.4 mg prn. Today, he reports his BP has been elevated at home. He also reports occasional chest pain that occurs approximately once per month. It is relieved by taking one nitroglycerin tablet. His BP and heart rate are 151/88 and 82, respectively, which have been confirmed twice in the past month. Which antihypertensive agent would you recommend for DL?

A BB, such as atenolol 25 mg QD, would be a good choice for DL due to the presence of stable angina. In addition to lowering blood pressure, BBs are excellent choices for prophylaxis of chest pain related to angina. Long-acting CCBs may also be used if he is intolerant of a BB or another agent is needed to control blood pressure.

References

1. The seventh report of the Joint National Committee on Prevention, Detection, Evaluation, and Treatment of High Blood Pressure. National Heart, Lung, and Blood Institute, National Institutes of Health, May 2003; NIH publication no. 03-5233.

2. The Writing Group of the PREMIER clinical trial. Effects of comprehensive lifestyle modification on blood pressure control. *JAMA*. 2003; 289:2083–93.

3. Appel LJ, Moore TJ, Obarzanek E et al. A clinical trial of the effects of dietary patterns on blood pressure. DASH Collaborative Research Group. *N Engl J Med*. 1997; 336:1117–24.

4. Kuczmarski RL, Flegal KM, Campbell SM et al. Increasing prevalence of overweight among US adults. *JAMA*. 1994; 272:205–11.

5. Chiang BN, Perlman, LV, Epstein FH. Overweight and hypertension. *Circulation*. 1969; 39:403–21.

6. Haffner S, Ferrannini E, Hazuda HP et al. Clustering of cardiovascular risk factors in confirmed prehypertensive individuals. *Hypertension*. 1992; 20:38–45.

7. Guagnano MT, Palitti VP, Mum R et al. Many factors can affect the prevalence of hypertension in obese patients: role of cuff size and type of obesity. *Panminerva Med*. 1998; 40(1):22–7.

8. Pouliot MC, Despres JP, Lemieux S et al. Waist circumference and abdominal sagittal diameter: best simple anthropometric indexes of abdominal visceral adipose tissue accumulation and related cardiovascular risk in men and women. *Am J Cardiol*. 1994; 73:460–8.

9. Despres JP, Lemieux I, Prud'homme D. Treatment of obesity: need to focus on high risk abdominally obese patients. *BMJ*. 2001; 322:716–20.

10. Reisin E, Abel R, Modan M et al. Effect of weight loss without salt restriction on the reduction of blood pressure in overweight hypertensive patients. *N Engl J Med*. 1978; 298:1–6.

11. Brenner BM, Garcia DL, Anderson S. Glomeruli and blood pressure. Less of one, more the other? *Am J Hypertens*. 1988; 1:335–47.

12. He J, Klag MJ, Caballero B et al. Plasma insulin levels and incidence of hypertension in African Americans and whites. *Arch Intern Med*. 1999; 159:498–503.

13. Obesity: preventing and managing the global epidemic. Report of a WHO consultation on obesity, Geneva, June 3–5, 1997. Geneva: World Health Organization; 1998.

14. 1999 World Health Organization–International Society of Hypertension Guidelines for the Management of Hypertension. *J Hypertens*. 1999; 17:151–83.

15. The Trials of Hypertension Prevention Collaborative Research Group. Effects of weight loss and sodium reduction intervention on blood pressure and hypertension incidence in overweight people with high-normal blood pressure. *Arch Intern Med*. 1997; 157:657–67.

16. Whelton PK, Appel LJ, Espeland MA et al. Sodium reduction and weight loss in the treatment of hypertension in older persons. *JAMA*. 1998; 279:839–46.

17. Neaton JD, Grimm RH Jr, Prineas RJ et al. Treatment of mild hypertension study. Final results. Treatment of Mild Hypertension Study Research Group. *JAMA*. 1993; 270:713–24.

18. Wadden TA, Foster GD. Behavioral treatment of obesity. *Med Clin North Am*. 2000; 84:441–61.

19. McGuire MT, Wing RR, Klem ML et al. Behavioral strategies of individuals who have maintained long-term weight losses. *Obes Res*. 1999; 7:334–41.

20. Lean ME, Han TS, Prvan T et al. Weight loss with high and low carbohydrate 1200 kcal diets in free living women. *Eur J Clin Nutr*. 1997; 51:243–8.

21. Executive summary of the third report of the National Cholesterol Education Program (NCEP) Expert Panel on Detection, Evaluation, and Treatment of High Blood Cholesterol in Adults. Treatment Panel III. *JAMA*. 2001; 285:2486–97.

22. Foster GD, Wyatt HR, Hill JO et al. A randomized trial of a low-carbohydrate diet for obesity. *N Engl J Med*. 2003; 348:2082–90.

23. Samaha FF, Iqbal N, Seshadri P et al. A low-carbohydrate as compared with a low-fat diet in severe obesity. *N Engl J Med*. 2003; 348:2074–81.

24. Bravata DM, Sanders L, Huang J et al. Efficacy and safety of low-carbohydrate diets: a systematic review. *JAMA*. 2003; 289:1837–50.

25. Clinical guidelines on the identification, evaluation, and treatment of overweight and obesity in adults—the evidence report. *Obes Res*. 1998; 6(Suppl 2):51S–209S.

26. Yanovski SZ, Yanovski JA. Obesity. *N Engl J Med*. 2002; 346:591–602.

27. 2000 Heart and Stroke Statistical Update. American Heart Association. Dallas, TX: American Heart Association; 1999.

28. Whelton SP, Chin A, Xin X et al. Effect of aerobic exercise on blood pressure: a meta-analysis of randomized, controlled trials. *Ann Intern Med*. 2002; 136:493–503.

29. Brown MD, Moore GE, Korytkowski MT et al. Improvement of insulin sensitivity by short-term exercise training in hypertensive African American women. *Hypertension*. 1997; 30:1549–53.

30. U.S. Department of Health and Human Services. Physical activity and health: a report of the Surgeon General. Atlanta, GA: Centers for Disease Control and Prevention, National Center for Chronic Disease Prevention and Health Promotion; 1996.

31. Thamer MA, Stewart KJ. Postmyocardial infarction care, cardiac rehabilitation, and physical conditioning. In: Principles of Ambulatory Medicine. Retford DC, ed. Baltimore: Williams and Wilkins; 1995:712.

32. Elliott P, Stamler J, Nichols R et al. Intersalt revisited: further analyses of 24 hour sodium excretion and blood pressure within and across populations. Intersalt Cooperative Research Group. *BMJ*. 1996; 312:1249–53.

33. Weinberger MH. Salt sensitivity of blood pressure in humans. *Hypertension*. 1996; 27:481–90.

34. Sacks FM, Svetkey LP, Vollmer WM et al. Effects on blood pressure of reduced dietary sodium and the Dietary Approaches to Stop Hypertension (DASH) diet. DASH–Sodium Collaborative Research Group. *N Engl J Med*. 2001; 344:3–10.

35. Mulrow C. Sound clinical advice for hypertensive patients. *Ann Intern Med*. 2001; 135:1084–6.

36. Dyer AR, Elliott P, Shipley M. Urinary electrolyte excretion in 24 hours and blood pressure in the INTERSALT study. The Intersalt Cooperative Research Group. *Am J Epidemiol.* 1994; 139:940–51.

37. Whelton PK, He J, Cutler JA et al. Effects of oral potassium on blood pressure. Meta-analysis of randomized controlled clinical trials. *JAMA.* 1997; 277:1624–32.

38. Campese VM. Calcium, parathyroid hormone, and blood pressure. *Am J Hypertens.* 1989; 2:34S–44S.

39. Cappuccio FP, Elliott P, Allender PS et al. Epidemiologic association between dietary calcium intake and blood pressure: a meta-analysis of published data. *Am J Epidemiol.* 1995; 142:935–45.

40. Allender PS, Cutler JA, Follmann D et al. Dietary calcium and blood pressure: a meta-analysis of randomized clinical trials. *Ann Intern Med.* 1996; 124:825–31.

41. Thun MJ, Peto R, Lopez AD et al. Alcohol consumption and mortality among middle-aged and elderly U.S. adults. *N Engl J Med.* 1997; 337:1705–14.

42. World Cancer Research Fund (WCRF) Panel. Diet, nutrition and the prevention of cancer: a global perspective. Washington, DC: World Cancer Research Fund; 1997.

43. McGinnis JM, Foege WH. Actual causes of death in the United States. *JAMA.* 1993; 270:2207–12.

44. Puddey IB, Beilin LJ, Rakic V. Alcohol, hypertension and the cardiovascular system: a critical appraisal. *Addict Biol.* 1997; 2:159–70.

45. Arkwright PD, Beilin LJ, Rouse I et al. Effects of alcohol use and other aspects of lifestyle on blood pressure levels and prevalence of hypertension in a working population. *Circulation.* 1982; 66:60–6.

46. MacMahon S. Alcohol consumption and hypertension. *Hypertension.* 1987; 9:111–21.

47. Puddey IB, Parker M, Beilen LJ et al. Effects of alcohol and caloric restrictions on blood pressure and serum lipids in overweight men. *Hypertension.* 1992; 20:533–41.

48. Frezza M, diPadova C, Pozzato G et al. High blood alcohol levels in women. The role of decreased gastric alcohol dehydrogenase activity and first-pass metabolism. *N Engl J Med.* 1990; 322:95–9.

49. Critchley JA, Capewell S. Mortality risk reduction associated with smoking cessation in patients with coronary heart disease: a systematic review. *JAMA.* 2003; 290:86–97.

50. Lee DH, Ha MH, Kim JR et al. Effects of smoking cessation on changes in blood pressure and incidence of hypertension: a 4-year follow up study. *Hypertension.* 2001; 37:194–8.

51. Halimi JM, Giraudeau B, Vol S et al. The risk of hypertension in men: direct and indirect effects of chronic smoking. *J Hypertens.* 2002; 20:187–93.

52. Oncken CA, White WB, Cooney JL et al. Impact of smoking cessation on ambulatory blood pressure and heart rate in postmenopausal women. *Am J Hypertens.* 2001; 14:942–9.

53. Minami J, Ishimitsu T, Matsuoka H. Is it time to regard cigarette smoking as a risk factor in the development of sustained hypertension? *Am J Hypertens.* 1999; 12:948–9.

54. Greenberg G, Thompson SG, Brennan PJ. The relationship between smoking and the response to antihypertensive treatment in mild hypertensives in the Medical Research Council's trial of treatment. *Int J Epidemiol.* 1987; 16:25–30.

55. Khoury Z, Comans P, Keren A et al. Effects of transdermal nicotine patches on ambulatory ECG monitoring findings: a double-blind study in healthy smokers. *Cardiovasc Drugs Ther.* 1996; 10:179–84.

56. A clinical practice guideline for treating tobacco use and dependence. U.S. Public Health Service Report. *JAMA.* 2000; 283:3244–54.

57. Klag MJ, Wang N, Meoni LA et al. Coffee intake and risk of hypertension: the Johns Hopkins precursors study. *Arch Intern Med.* 2002; 162:657–62.

58. Hartley TR, Sung BH, Pincomb GA et al. Hypertension risk status and effect of caffeine on blood pressure. *Hypertension.* 2000; 36(1):137–41.

59. Rakic V, Burke V, Beilin LJ. Effects of coffee on ambulatory blood pressure in older men and women: a randomized controlled trial. *Hypertension.* 1999; 33(3):869–73.

60. Guideline Committee of the European Society of Hypertension–European Society of Cardiology. 2003 European Society of Hypertension–European Society of Cardiology guidelines for the management of arterial hypertension. *J Hypertens.* 2003; 21:1011–53.

61. Major outcomes in high-risk hypertensive patients randomized to angiotensin-converting enzyme inhibitor or calcium channel blocker vs diuretic. The Antihypertensive and Lipid-Lowering Treatment to Prevent Heart Attack Trial (ALLHAT) Collaborative Research Group. *JAMA.* 2002; 288:2981–97.

62. Dahlof B, Devereux RB, Kjeldsen SE et al. Cardiovascular morbidity and mortality in the Losartan Intervention For Endpoint reduction in hypertension study (LIFE): a randomised trial against atenolol. *Lancet.* 2002; 359:995–1003.

63. Hansson L, Hedner T, Johansen P et al. Randomised trial of effects of calcium antagonists compared with diuretics and BBs on cardiovascular morbidity and mortality in hypertension: the Nordic Diltiazem (NORDIL) study. *Lancet.* 2000; 345:359–65.

64. Prevention of stroke by antihypertensive drug treatment in older persons with isolated systolic hypertension. Final results of the Systolic Hypertension in the Elderly Program (SHEP). SHEP Cooperative Research Group. *JAMA.* 1991; 265:3255–64.

65. Hansson L, Lindholm LH, Ekbom T et al. Randomised trial of old and new antihypertensive drugs in elderly patients: cardiovascular mortality and morbidity in the Swedish Trial in Old Patients with Hypertension-2 study. *Lancet.* 1999; 354:1751–6.

66. Wing LM, Reid CM, Ryan P et al. A comparison of outcomes with angiotensin-converting-enzyme inhibitors and diuretics for hypertension in the elderly. *N Engl J Med.* 2003; 348:583–92.

67. Staessen JA, Fagard R, Thijs L et al. Randomised double-blind comparison of placebo and active treatment for older patients with isolated systolic hypertension. Systolic Hypertension in Europe (Syst-Eur) Trial Investigators. *Lancet.* 1997; 350:757–64.

68. Update on the 1987 Task Force Report on High Blood

Pressure in Children and Adolescents: a working group report from the National High Blood Pressure Education Program. National High Blood Pressure Education Program Working Group on Hypertension Control in Children and Adolescents. *Pediatrics*. 1995; 98:649–58.

69. National High Blood Pressure Education Program Working Group report on hypertension in the elderly. National High Blood Pressure Education Program Working Group. *Hypertension*. 1994; 23:275–85.

70. Medical Research Council trial of treatment of hypertension in older adults; principal results. MRC Working Party. *BMJ*. 1992; 304:405–12.

71. Dahlof B, Lindholm LH, Hansson L et al. Morbidity and mortality in the Swedish Trial in Old Patients with Hypertension (STOP-Hypertension). *Lancet*. 1991; 338:1281–5.

72. Liu L, Wang JG, Gong L et al. Comparison of active treatment and placebo in older Chinese patients with isolated systolic hypertension. Systolic Hypertension in China (Syst-China) Collaborative Group. *J Hypertens*. 1998; 16:1823–9.

73. Gueyffier F, Boutitie F, Boissel JP et al. Effect of antihypertensive drug treatment on cardiovascular outcomes in women and men. A meta-analysis of individual patient data from randomized, controlled trials. The INDANA Investigators. *Ann Intern Med*. 1997; 126:761–7.

74. The sixth report of the Joint National Committee on Prevention, Detection, Evaluation, and Treatment of High Blood Pressure. National Heart, Lung, and Blood Institute, National Institutes of Health, November 1997; NIH publication no. 98-4080.

75. Wright JT Jr, Bakris G, Greene T et al. Effect of blood pressure lowering and antihypertensive drug class on progression of hypertensive kidney disease: results from the AASK trial. *JAMA*. 2002; 288:2421–31.

76. Estacio RO, Jeffers BW, Hiatt WR et al. The effect of nisoldipine as compared with enalapril on cardiovascular outcomes in patients with non-insulin-dependent diabetes and hypertension. *N Engl J Med*. 1998; 338:645–52.

77. Major cardiovascular events in hypertensive patients randomized to doxazosin vs chlorthalidone: the Antihypertensive and Lipid-Lowering Treatment to Prevent Heart Attack Trial (ALLHAT). Antihypertensive Therapy and Lipid Lowering Heart Attack Trial (ALLHAT) Collaborative Research Group. *JAMA*. 2000; 283:1967–75.

78. Hansson L, Lindholm LH, Niskanen L et al. Effect of angiotensin-converting-enzyme inhibition compared with conventional therapy on cardiovascular morbidity and mortality in hypertension: the Captopril Prevention Project (CAPPP) randomised trial. *Lancet*. 1999; 353:611–6.

79. Tatti P, Pahor M, Byington RP et al. Outcome results of the Fosinopril Versus Amlodipine Cardiovascular Events Randomized Trial (FACET) in patients with hypertension and NIDDM. *Diabetes Care*. 1998; 21:597–603.

80. Hansson L, Zanchetti A, Carruthers SG et al. Effects of intensive blood-pressure lowering and low-dose aspirin in patients with hypertension: principal results of the Hypertension Optimal Treatment (HOT) randomised trial. HOT Study Group. *Lancet*. 1998; 351:1755–62.

81. Brown MJ, Palmer CR, Castaigne A et al. Morbidity and mortality in patients randomised to double-blind treatment with a long-acting calcium-channel blocker or diuretic in the International Nifedipine GITS study. Intervention as a Goal in Hypertension Treatment (INSIGHT). *Lancet*. 2000; 345:366–72.

82. Borhani NO, Mercuri M, Borhani PA et al. Final outcome results of the multicenter isradipine diuretic atherosclerosis study (MIDAS). A randomized controlled trial. *JAMA*. 1996; 276:785–91.

83. Braunwald E, Antman EM, Beasley JW et al. ACC/AHA 2002 guideline update for the management of patients with unstable angina and non-ST-segment elevation myocardial infarction. *J Am Coll Cardiol*. 2002; 40:1366–74.

84. Braunwald E, Antman EM, Beasley JW et al. ACC/AHA guidelines for the management of patients with unstable angina and non-ST-segment elevation myocardial infarction. A report of the American College of Cardiology/American Heart Association Task Force on Practice Guidelines (Committee on the Management of Patients with Unstable Angina). *J Am Coll Cardiol*. 2000; 36:970–1062.

85. Gibbons RJ, Chatterjee K, Daley J et al. ACC/AHA/ACP-ASIM guidelines for the management of patients with chronic stable angina: a report of the American College of Cardiology/American Heart Association Task Force on Practice Guidelines. *J Am Coll Cardiol*. 1999; 33:2092–197.

86. Lewis EJ, Hunsicker LG, Bain RP et al. The effect of angiotensin-converting-enzyme inhibition on diabetic nephropathy. Collaborative Study Group. *N Engl J Med*. 1993; 329:1456–62.

87. Efficacy of atenolol and captopril in reducing risk of macrovascular and microvascular complications in type 2 diabetes: UKPDS 39. UK Prospective Diabetes Study Group. *BMJ*. 1998; 317:713–20.

88. Ravid M, Brosh D, Levi Z et al. Use of enalapril to attenuate decline in renal function in normotensive, normoalbuminuric patients with type 2 diabetes mellitus. A randomized, controlled trial. *Ann Intern Med*. 1998; 128:982–8.

89. Sano T, Kawamura T, Matsumae H et al. Effects of long-term enalapril treatment on persistent microalbuminuria in well-controlled hypertensive and normotensive NIDDM patients. *Diabetes Care*. 1994; 17: 420–4.

90. Yusuf S, Sleight P, Pogue J et al. Effects of an angiotensin-converting-enzyme inhibitor, ramipril, on cardiovascular events in high-risk patients. The Heart Outcomes Prevention Evaluation Study Investigators. *N Engl J Med*. 2000; 342:145–53.

91. Lewis EJ, Hunsicker LG, Clarke WR et al. Renoprotective effect of the angiotensin-receptor antagonist irbesartan in patients with nephropathy due to type 2 diabetes. Collaborative Study Group. *N Engl J Med*. 2001; 345:851–60.

92. Garg R, Yusuf S. Overview of randomized trials of an-

giotensin-converting enzyme inhibitors on mortality and morbidity in patients with heart failure. Collaborative Group on ACE Inhibitor Trials. *JAMA.* 1995; 273:1450–6.

93. American Diabetes Association. Treatment of hypertension in adults with diabetes. *Diabetes Care.* 2003; 26(Suppl 1):S80–2.

94. National Kidney Foundation Guideline. K/DOQI clinical practice guidelines for chronic kidney disease: evaluation, classification, and stratification. Kidney Disease Outcome Quality Initiative. *Am J Kidney Dis.* 2002; 39(Suppl 2):S1–246.

95. Packer M, Bristow MR, Cohn JN et al. The effect of carvedilol on morbidity and mortality in patients with chronic heart failure. *N Engl J Med.* 1996; 334:1349–55.

96. The cardiac insufficiency bisoprolol study II (CIBIS-II): a randomised trial. *Lancet.* 1999; 353:9–13.

97. Hjalmarson A, Goldstein S, Fagerberg B et al. Effects of controlled-release metoprolol on total mortality, hospitalizations, and well-being in patients with heart failure: the Metoprolol CR/XL Randomized Intervention Trial in congestive heart failure (MERIT-HF). MERIT-HF Study Group. *JAMA.* 2000; 283:1295–302.

98. Dargie HJ. Effect of carvedilol on outcome after myocardial infarction in patients with left-ventricular dysfunction: the CAPRICORN randomised trial. *Lancet.* 2001; 357:1385–90.

99. Hunt SA, Baker DW, Chin MH et al. ACC/AHA guidelines for the evaluation and management of chronic heart failure in the adult: executive summary. *J Am Coll Cardiol.* 2001; 38:2101–13.

100. Cohn JN, Tognoni G. A randomized trial of the angiotensin-receptor blocker valsartan in chronic heart failure. *N Engl J Med.* 2001; 345:1667–75.

101. Pitt B, Zannad F, Remme WJ et al. The effect of spironolactone on morbidity and mortality in patients with severe heart failure. Randomized Aldactone Evaluation Study Investigators. *N Engl J Med.* 1999; 341:709–17.

102. Hennekens CH, Albert CM, Godfried SL et al. Adjunctive drug therapy of acute myocardial infarction—evidence from clinical trials. *N Engl J Med.* 1996; 335:1660–7.

103. Pitt B, Remme W, Zannad F et al. Eplerenone, a selective aldosterone blocker, in patients with left ventricular dysfunction after myocardial infarction. *N Engl J Med.* 2003; 348:1309–21.

104. Black HR, Elliott WJ, Grandits G et al. Principal results of the Controlled Onset Verapamil Investigation of Cardiovascular End Points (CONVINCE) trial. *JAMA.* 2003; 289:2073–82.

105. Maschio G, Alberti D, Janin G et al. Effect of the angiotensin-converting enzyme inhibitor benazepril on the progression of chronic renal insufficiency. Angiotensin-Converting-Enzyme Inhibition in Progressive Renal Insufficiency Study Group. *N Engl J Med.* 1996; 334:939–45.

106. Randomised placebo-controlled trial of effect of ramipril on decline in glomerular filtration rate and risk of terminal renal failure in proteinuric, non-diabetic nephropathy. The GISEN (Gruppo Italiano di Studi Epidemiologici in Nefrologia) Group. *Lancet.* 1997; 349:1857–63.

107. Randomised trial of a perindopril-based blood-pressure-lowering regimen among 6105 individuals with previous stroke or transient ischaemic attack. PROGRESS Collaborative Group. *Lancet.* 2001; 358: 1033–41.

108. Yee GC, McGuire TR. Pharmacokinetic drug interactions with cyclosporin. *Clin Pharmacokinet.* 1990; 19:400–15.

109. Mangano DT, Layug EL, Wallace A et al. Effect of atenolol on mortality and cardiovascular morbidity after noncardiac surgery. Multicenter Study of Perioperative Ischemia Research Group. *N Engl J Med.* 1996; 335:1713–20.

110. Savage PJ, Pressel SL, Curb JD et al. Influence of long-term, low-dose, diuretic-based, antihypertensive therapy on glucose, lipid, uric acid, and potassium levels in older men and women with isolated systolic hypertension: The Systolic Hypertension in the Elderly Program. SHEP Cooperative Research Group. *Arch Intern Med.* 1998; 158:741–51.

111. Sibai BM. Treatment of hypertension in pregnant women. *N Engl J Med.* 1996; 335:257–65.

Appendix 6-1.
Examples of Sites for Smoking Cessation on the Internet

Tobacco Cessation Guideline

http://www.surgeongeneral.gov/tobacco

New findings about the latest drugs and counseling techniques for treating tobacco use and dependence.

Free Web-based Smoking Cessation Study

https://stopsmoking.ucsf.edu/pages/#

This is the site for a UCSF research study to determine what proportion of smokers can quit using the Web.

WebMD—Smoking Cessation: No Butts About It!

http://my.webmd.com/roundtable_topic/49

8 week stop-smoking program with online discussion from participants.

Mediconsult.com: Smoking Cessation, Quit Smoking Information

http://www.mediconsult.com/mc/mcsite.nsf/conditionnav/

Smoking Cessation, Stop Smoking health resources from Mediconsult.com for patients and professionals, educational material, news, drug information, journal articles, community, support. Site pulls together information from other sources.

A Guide to Smoking Cessation

http://www.geocities.com/CapeCanaveral/Lab/1246/

For people wanting to quit smoking, for physicians and students who want to help their patients or just want to gain more knowledge.

Smoking Cessation by About.com

http://quitsmoking.about.com

Find help you need to kick the habit and stay smoke-free. Fight your nicotine addiction, and keep your hands busy after quitting.

QuitsmokingMD

http://www.wellmd. com/quitsmokingmd.htm

Physician supervised interactive smoking cessation programs, smoking news, and information.

Appendix 6-2.
Indigent Care Drug Therapy Sites

1. http://www.needymeds.com
   NeedyMeds.com

   Many pharmaceutical manufacturers have special programs to assist people who cannot afford to buy the drugs they need. One problem is that it is often hard to learn about these programs. This site makes this information easily accessible.

   Each company has its own program with its special requirements, forms, and procedures. Some companies have different programs for different drugs. There is no central clearinghouse for obtaining up-to-date information about these programs or the drugs themselves.

2. http://www.rxbenefits.com/discount/index.html
   Prescription Benefits, Inc

   Pharmacy services offered include:

   - AdvanceRx.com™—refill AdvanceRx.com™ prescriptions
   - AdvanceRx.com™ order form—for new prescriptions
   - Order tracking—track AdvanceRx.com™ refill order status
   - Pharmacy locator—search for a pharmacy
   - Ask a pharmacist—email questions to a pharmacist
   - Nonprescription products—shop for drugstore needs
   - More pharmacy services—order Rite Aid or drugstore.com prescriptions and more

3. http://www.phrma.org/searchcures/dpdpap/pa99.pdf

   Directory of prescription drug patient assistance programs

   For a printout of the entire program with applicable companies participating, see this site; additional copies of this directory can be obtained by calling (800) 762-4636.

   The research-based pharmaceutical industry has had a long-standing tradition of providing prescription medicines free of charge to physicians whose patients might not otherwise have access to necessary medicines. To make it easier for physicians to identify the growing number of programs available for needy patients, member companies of the Pharmaceutical Research and Manufacturers of America (PhRMA) created this directory. It lists company programs that provide drugs to physicians whose patients could not otherwise afford them. The programs are listed alphabetically by company. Under the entry for each program is information about how to make a request for assistance, what prescription medicines are covered, and basic eligibility criteria.

4. http://www.rxhope.com

   RxHope.com is the only patient assistance Internet initiative financially supported by PhRMA and participating pharmaceutical companies.

   RxHope.com began as a grassroots effort of the Patient Assistance Managers and Directors of the PhRMA-member companies and has grown into the leading Internet-based patient assistance and sampling web portal in the pharmaceutical industry. Each patient assistance request form has been custom designed to the pharmaceutical company's rules engine. RxHope.com does not approve or deny requests nor does it take delivery or ship product; it merely removes the time and costs of these programs by web-enabling labor-intensive paperwork onto the physician's computer.

   For patients, physicians, patient advocates, and pharmaceutical companies, the benefits are substantial:

   - Faster processing
   - Physicians requesting samples and their qualified applicants can receive pharmaceutical products quickly versus the weeks, or even months, it currently takes to process these requests.
   - Less time resources required
   - The physician's office completes the requisition process in just a few minutes. The request is then electronically forwarded to the pharmaceutical company for processing.
   - Financial savings
   - Less money spent on postage, printed material, opening and sorting requests, and other time-consuming tasks. There is no charge to the patient, physician, or patient advocate for these services

   RxHope.com also offers an Assistance Finder, which matches patient information against other available federal, state, and charitable prescription drug programs. RxHope.com is a privately held company located in Hackettstown, NJ; direct questions or comments to:

   RxHope.com
   254 Mountain Avenue
   Building B, Suite 303
   Hackettstown, NJ 07840
   Telephone: (908) 850-8004
   Fax: (908) 850-8269
   email: customerservice@rxhope.com

5. http://www.medicare.gov/AssistancePrograms/home.asp

   This section provides information on programs that offer discounts or free medication to individuals in need. To find information on prescription drug assistance programs, Medicare managed care plans, and Medigap plans that offer prescription drug coverage, fill in the form. For more information on prescription drug coverage, look at frequently asked questions and answers.

Chapter 7:

Education of Ambulatory Hypertensive Patients

Beth Bryles Phillips

Clinical Highlights

- What are key elements that should be communicated to the patient with hypertension?
- What types of monitors are more likely to produce reliable home blood pressure measurements?
- What are the general recommendations for home blood pressure monitoring?
- What resources are available for educating hypertensive patients?

In order to achieve optimal control of blood pressure (BP) and subsequently minimize adverse outcomes associated with hypertension, the health care provider and patient must work as a team. Patients should have a clear understanding of the significance of hypertension, its treatment, and adverse consequences of uncontrolled hypertension so that they can make informed decisions about their health. Additionally, patients should be actively involved and interested in how they can participate in improving their health. Patients may participate in the treatment of hypertension and possibly improve their own outcomes by implementing lifestyle modifications, avoiding therapies that may increase their BP, and monitoring their own BP outside of the office. Because there is so much information to learn and comprehend on this topic, ongoing encouragement and reinforcement for patients is essential.

Comprehensive Education

To successfully educate the ambulatory patient about hypertension, several topics should be discussed. Providing patients with written information is a good way to reinforce the principles verbally discussed. Several excellent resources exist providing written patient information that can be given to patients at no charge. Other very good resources, such as educational videos, are available that can be purchased for patient use. (These resources are discussed in more detail in the Resources section at the end of the chapter.) Included

in **Appendix 7-1** is a comprehensive educational handout on hypertension available from the National Heart, Lung, and Blood Institute (NHLBI). Thorough patient education on hypertension should include the following topics:

- Overview: Patients should have an understanding of what hypertension is, its prevalence, why it is dangerous, and how it is detected. An explanation of hypertension, or high BP, should be given to patients. Patients should understand that, although it is a common disease (affecting approximately 25% of the American population), the adverse consequences of inadequately controlled blood pressure are serious.

- Benefits, risks, and management options: Patients should understand the asymptomatic nature of hypertension, the risks of uncontrolled hypertension, and how to control BP. They should recognize the signs of target organ damage (e.g., myocardial infarction, stroke, heart failure, renal failure, and retinopathies) and the risk factors for cardiovascular disease, such as age, smoking, diabetes, hypercholesterolemia, and obesity. They should also be encouraged to lead a healthy lifestyle (e.g., losing weight, limiting the amount of salt and fat in their diet, increasing potassium and calcium in the diet, exercising, limiting alcohol to two or less drinks daily, and refraining from cigarette smoking). The NHLBI publication, "Lowering Your Blood Pressure" (included in Appendix 7-1), provides several examples of moderate exercise in which patients should engage. Additionally, it also provides several tips to reduce dietary sodium and other healthy dietary suggestions.

- Stress and social support: A discussion on proper social support and encouragement should be included, especially as lifestyle changes can be very difficult for some patients.

- Exercise and activity: Regular exercise and activity can assist in lowering blood pressure and specifically help in achieving weight reduction goals. Patients should be encouraged to perform moderate-level exercise for 30 minutes at least several times a week. For patients who have physical limitations to exercise, a referral to a physical therapist may be appropriate.

- Medications (including over-the-counter or OTC and herbal therapies): Patients should be thoroughly educated about the antihypertensive medications they are taking, including the names of their medications, doses, proper use, administration, and storage; common adverse effects; and drug interactions. Certain OTC, alternative, and prescription medications can adversely affect blood pressure. Some medications and factors that can raise blood pressure are listed in **Table 7-1**. Additionally, a list of drug–herb interactions specifically in regard to antihypertensive medications is given in **Table 7-2**. Patients should be encouraged to report all OTC and alternative therapy use to their health care providers. Any additional therapies should be checked for drug–drug or drug–disease state interactions. Adherence to the antihypertensive drug therapy regimen should also be stressed. Patients should be encouraged to use a medication box if appropriate to assist medication administration. Patients should keep a list of all medications (including antihypertensive medications) with them at all times.

- Monitoring and use of results: Patients should understand how blood pressure is measured and how often it should be monitored. An explanation of systolic and diastolic blood pressures will help them understand what is being measured. They should also be aware of their recommended blood pressure goals (e.g., target blood pressure less than 140/90 mm Hg for patients with uncomplicated hypertension). A record of home blood pressure recordings should be brought to each visit, if recommended.

- Prevention, detection, and treatment of complications related to uncontrolled hypertension: The ultimate goal in treating hypertension is to prevent adverse outcomes, such as cardiovascular, cerebrovascular, and renal diseases and retinopathy. Patients should be able to recognize the signs and symptoms of target organ damage and how the risk of developing these complications can be minimized.

- Behavior change strategies, goal setting, risk factor reduction, and problem solving: The appropriate management of hypertension will require lifestyle modification for most patients. The presence of modifiable risk factors for cardiovascular disease, such as hypertension, hyperlipidemia, smoking, diabetes, obesity, and physical inactivity, should be identified for each patient. Once these factors have been determined, patients should set goals for themselves to abolish or minimize these risk factors. For example, an obese patient could set a goal of initially reducing total body weight by 10%. A smoker may evaluate various methods of smoking cessation and set a "quit date" to stop smoking.

- Preconception care, pregnancy: Women with child-bearing potential who are taking antihypertensive medication should be educated on proper methods of contraception as some antihypertensive agents may be teratogenic. If a woman becomes or is planning to become pregnant, she should consult her obstetrician.

- Use of health care systems and community resources: Patients should be made aware of resources for hypertensive patients available in their community.

Drug Interactions

There are a number of medications, substances, and alternative therapies that may contribute to elevations in blood pressure. A list of common factors that may increase blood pressure can be found in Table 7-1. Health care providers should be aware of these factors and screen for them as appropriate. A complete medical history, including the use of alternative therapies and substances, should be taken for all patients. Because many patients do not readily share information about alternative therapy use with their health care providers, it is important to periodically ask patients about their use. Patients should be asked to notify their health care provider before initiating therapy with a new alternative medication. Additionally, patients should be aware of OTC medications such as decongestants or non-

Table 7-1.

Factors That Can Adversely Affect Blood Pressure[1]

Medications	Substances	Alternative Therapies
Adrenal steroids	Alcohol	Burdock
General anesthetics	Amphetamines	Ephedra
Noradrenergic or serotonergic appetite suppressants	Cannabis	Ginger
Cyclosporine	Cocaine	Goldenseal
Decongestants		Licorice
Disulfiram		Panax ginseng
Epoetin (erythropoietin)		Siberian ginseng
Monoamine oxidase inhibitors		Yohimbe
Nonsteroidal anti-inflammatory drugs (NSAIDs)		
Oral contraceptives		
Abrupt discontinuation of specific antihypertensive agents (i.e., beta-blockers or clonidine)		
Venlafaxine		

Table 7-2.

Drug–Herb Interactions between Antihypertensive Agents and Alternative Therapies

Drug	Alternative Therapy	Interaction
Antihypertensive agents	Devil's claw, European mistletoe	May increase the effect of anti-hypertensive by causing hypotension
Antihypertensive agents	Fish oils, Stinging nettle (above ground parts), yohimbe	May interfere with blood pressure control
Antihypertensive agents	Ginger, goldenseal, licorice	May decrease the effectiveness of antihypertensive by increasing blood pressure
Calcium channel blockers	St. John's wort	May interfere with metabolism of CCB through cytochrome P-450 3A4 and p-glycoprotein
Calcium channel blockers	Grapefruit juice (large quantities)	May interfere with metabolism of CCB through cytochrome P-450 3A4
Potassium-depleting diuretics	Aloe latex, cascara, gossypol, licorice	May increase potassium loss
Reserpine	St. John's wort	May antagonize the effects of reserpine
Thiazide diuretics	Gingko leaf extract	May increase blood pressure when used with thiazides

steroidal anti-inflammatory drugs (NSAIDs) that can raise blood pressure.

Home Monitoring of Blood Pressure

Monitoring blood pressure outside of the health care provider's office and particularly patient ownership of sphygmomanometers has become more popular. Home blood pressure (HBP) monitoring may be helpful in determining the blood pressure without the anxiety of measuring it in a health care setting and in evaluating the effect of antihypertensive therapy.[2]

There are a variety of manual and digital devices patients may purchase for HBP monitoring. Of the manual devices, aneroid sphygmomanometers are more popular for home use. They are relatively inexpensive and reliable, although they may become less accurate over time and recalibration must be performed. Mercury sphygmomanometers are more accurate. However, environmental concerns have limited their use in the home.

Electronic devices measure blood pressure using either the auscultatory or oscillometric method. Both methods correlate well with manual determinations of BP. However, excess noise may affect BP measurements determined by the auscultatory method and excess movement may alter measurements determined by the oscillometric method. Most electronic devices now utilize the oscillometric method of measuring BP.[3] One type of electronic device, the finger BP monitor, is not reliable and should not be recommended for use in the home.[4] Factors that may affect the accuracy of finger BP monitors include peripheral vasoconstriction, measuring BP at a site more distal than the upper arm, and variability of measurement related to position of the extremity.[5] Another alternative method for HBP is using an electronic wrist device. Although this device may yield reliable measurements with appropriate use, the accuracy is highly dependent on arm position. The monitor must be held at the level of the heart in order to obtain reliable measurements.[3] Without proper instruction and ongoing monitoring of patient use, it may be difficult to determine if HBP measurements determined by this method are accurate.

HBP monitoring is viewed favorably by many professional societies, including the Joint National Committee on the Prevention, Detection, Evaluation, and Treatment of High Blood Pressure.[6] Recommendations for HBP monitoring have been published by the American Society of Hypertension[2] and the Canadian Coalition for High Blood Pressure Prevention and Control.[7] According to the American Society of Hypertension Ad Hoc Panel, HBP monitoring is generally recommended for most hypertensive patients for the following reasons: (1) it may help distinguish between white coat and sustained hypertension; (2) it may help assess the effect of antihypertensive therapy; (3) it may improve patient adherence to drug therapy and

lifestyle modifications; and (4) it may reduce costs.[2] Additionally, some data suggest that HBP monitoring may correlate better with target organ damage than office measurements.[3] Patients who may not be candidates for HBP monitoring are those with irregular heart rhythms (e.g., atrial fibrillation) and those with morbid obesity.

There are several general recommendations for patients who plan to monitor blood pressure at home. It is advisable that patients obtain a sphygmomanometer meeting the Association for the Advancement of Medical Instrumentation (AAMI) and/or British Hypertension Society Standards. These monitors have demonstrated accuracy and compliance with strict standards. A list of such devices can be found in **Table 7-3**. Several of the monitors listed in Table 7-3 can be found at medical supply stores or on the Internet. Many models cost between $50 and $100. Patients should also be asked to record measurements in the morning and evening, including both work and non-work days. The frequency of measurements may vary and should be based upon the patient's clinical situation. For example, a patient with newly diagnosed hypertension or BP that is difficult to control may be asked to record several readings per week. A patient with stable, controlled hypertension may not need to perform HBP monitoring as often.[2] If patients report difficulty in measuring HBP or if HBP measurements repeatedly are in disagreement with office BP, it may be helpful to review the monitor and technique used for HBP monitoring. **Table 7-4** lists several factors which may lead to discrepant HBP measurements.

Several studies have been conducted in an effort to determine optimal HBP measurements. Although the methodology of the studies varied, there seems to be general agreement that optimal HBP values are less than those acceptable by office mea-

---

Table 7-3.

Home Blood Pressure Monitors Meeting Association for the Advancement of Medical Instrumentation (AAMI) and/or British Hypertension Society Standards[3]

Instrument	Model	Manufacturer
Assure	A30, W20	Becton, Dickinson & Co; Franklin Lakes, NJ
A & D	UA-767, UA-767PC	A & D Co, Ltd; Tokyo, Japan
Instromedix QD	—	ALARIS Medical Systems, Inc; San Diego, CA
Omron	HEM-706, 705CP, 711, 722c, 713c, and 403c	Omron Healthcare, Inc; Vernon Hills, IL
Terumo	ES-H51	Terumo Medical Corp; Somerset, NJ

Table 7-4.

Factors Commonly Associated with Erroneous Home Blood Pressure Measurements*

Factor	Mercury Devices	Aneroid Devices	Automatic Devices
Incorrect placement of bladder cuff	+	+	+
Incorrect cuff size (cuff that is too small may give falsely elevated measurements)	+	+	+
Inaccurate pressure gauge		+	+
Difficulty in reading gauge due to visual problems		+	
Inadequate stethoscope	+	+	
Inappropriate placement of stethoscope or transducer (not over brachial artery)	+	+	+
Hearing loss resulting in difficulty determining measurement	+	+	
Rapid cuff deflation resulting in estimation of Korotkoff sounds	+	+	
Measurement of Korotkoff IV sound	+	+	+
Inadequate number of readings	+	+	+
Inaccurate recording of measurements	+	+	+
Leaking bulbs, valves, or hoses	+	+	+
Underinflation of cuff (resulting in systolic measurement that is too low)	+	+	
Atrial fibrillation			+
Rounding of last numerical digit in measurement		+	

*Adapted and reprinted with permission from Yarrows SA, Julius S, Pickering TG. Home blood pressure monitoring. *Arch Intern Med.* 2000; 160:1251–7.

surements. Some experts recommend that the optimal upper limit values for HBP measurements are no higher than 130/80 to 135/85 mm Hg.[3]

Educational Approaches

There are many factors that affect the proper educational approach to a particular patient, including illiteracy, age, education, and physical or mental impairment. Visual aids should be substituted for written information when educating illiterate patients about hypertension. For example, a color-coded medication schedule or a picture chart showing medications and the time of day they are to be taken may be used. Elderly patients who have cataracts, macular degeneration, or other visual difficulties may need written information in large print so it is easier to read. Patients with a low educational level may have difficulty understanding medication directions or comprehending written information. It is important to prepare written information with an easier reading level for these patients and always provide written medication instructions that are easily understood.

Conversely, highly educated patients, especially those in the health care field, will appreciate when more medical jargon is used in communicating hypertension information. However, care should be taken not to omit or shorten the information normally given to other hypertensive patients due to the assumption the patient is already aware of the information. Some patients may have mental or physical impairments that limit the ability to care for themselves. These patients often have a caregiver who assists with their health care needs. In these instances, it is important that the caregiver has proper instructions needed to properly care for the patient. For example, the caregiver should have a list of the patient's medications with instructions on when and how to administer them.

Resources

Appropriately educating hypertensive patients about their disease is extremely important. Several patient-related factors may warrant varied educational approaches. Fortunately, a wealth of educational resources for the hypertensive patient exists.

Many very good resources are available at no charge, while others may have a fee associated with them. Many organizations devoted to the treatment of hypertension offer educational materials for patients. A summary of several resources and a description of available materials are included in **Table 7-5**. The reader should also be aware that resources also exist providing unproven information

---

Table 7-5.
Educational Resources

American Heart Association (AHA)

www.americanheart.org

http://www.americanheart.org/
    Heart_and_Stroke_A_Z_Guide/hbp.html

Professional Resources

The AHA website offers numerous resources for professionals, including professional guidelines and statements.

Patient Education Material

The AHA offers Lifestyle Information Sheets on the following topics related to hypertension:

- High blood pressure
- Smoking
- Physical activity
- Nutrition and weight management

AHA

http://www.americanheart.org/Patient_Information/

(800) 611-6082

Patient Education Material

Answers by Heart. A kit containing 53 sheets of patient education material that can be photocopied for patients. Topics include a wide range of cardiovascular subjects. Handouts available in Spanish also.

Patient Education Video Series. A series of videos concerning cardiovascular wellness, conditions, and procedures. Videos are available in Spanish also. Videos specifically pertaining to hypertension include:

- How to Monitor Your Blood Pressure
- Hypertension

American Society of Hypertension (ASH)

http://www.ash-us.org/2001a/hypertensionfaq.html

Patient Education Material

ASH offers a patient information guide, "Understanding Hypertension." This guide is available in portable document format (pdf).

National Heart, Lung, and Blood Institute (NHLBI)

www.nhlbi.nih.gov

http://www.nhlbi.nih.gov/health/public/heart/
    index.htm

Professional Resources

The NHLBI offers guidelines, reports, statements, quick reference guides, and slide kits for use by the health care professional.

- Working Group Report on High Blood Pressure in Pregnancy
- Statement from the National High Blood Pressure Education Program Coordinating Committee Regarding the Consumption of Dietary Salt
- Workshop on Sodium and Blood Pressure
- Your Guide to Lowering High Blood Pressure
- The seventh report of the Joint National Committee (JNC 7) on High Blood Pressure
- JNC 7 Quick Reference Card
- Report on High Blood Pressure in Children and Adolescents
- Implementing Recommendations for Dietary Salt Reduction
- Report on Primary Prevention of High Blood Pressure
- Working Group Report on Ambulatory Blood Pressure Monitoring
- Working Group Report on Hypertension in Diabetes
- National High Blood Pressure Education Program (NHBPEP)
- High Blood Pressure Information Slide Sets

Patient Education Material

The NHLBI offers several educational sheets that can be printed and given to patients. Many handouts are available in pdf.

- Your Guide to Lowering High Blood Pressure (Interactive Web Site)
- Facts about the DASH Diet
- High Blood Pressure in Pregnancy
- Facts about Lowering Blood Pressure
- DASHing with Less Salt
- How to Prevent High Blood Pressure
- Controlling High Blood Pressure: A Guide for Older Women
- Facts about Heart Disease and Women: Preventing and Controlling High Blood Pressure
- Controlling High Blood Pressure: A Woman's Guide
- Stay Young at Heart Recipes
- National High Blood Pressure Education Program

Key Points for Patients

- Patients should have an understanding of what hypertension is, its prevalence, why it is dangerous, and how it is detected.

- Patients should be monitored for factors that may cause an increase in blood pressure or a loss of blood pressure control.

- Home blood pressure monitoring may be helpful in determining the presence of white coat hypertension, assessing the effect of antihypertensive therapy, improving patient adherence, correlating with target organ damage, and reducing costs.

- Patients should receive guidance for appropriate choice of a home blood pressure monitor, technique in determining home blood pressure measurements, and frequency of monitoring.

- The educational approach to the patient with hypertension should take into account factors such as illiteracy, age, education, and physical or mental impairment.

- Several informational resources exist for patients with hypertension. Patients should be directed toward accurate material that is easy to comprehend.

---

about hypertension. The reader should evaluate hypertension information before providing it to the patient.

References

1. O'Rorke JE, Richardson WS. Evidence based management of hypertension: What to do when blood pressure is difficult to control. *BMJ.* 2001; 322:1229–32.

2. Pickering T. Recommendations for the use of home (self) and ambulatory blood pressure monitoring. *Am J Hypertens.* 1995; 9:1–11.

3. Yarrows SA, Julius S, Pickering TG. Home blood pressure monitoring. *Arch Intern Med.* 2000; 160:1251–7.

4. Nesselrod JM, Flacco VA, Phillips KM et al. Accuracy of automated finger blood pressure devices. *Fam Med.* 1995; 28:182–92.

5. O'Brien E, Beevers G, Lip GY. Blood pressure measurement. Part IV–automated sphygmomanometry: self blood pressure measurement. *BMJ.* 2001; 322:1167–70.

6. The seventh report of the Joint National Committee on Prevention, Detection, Evaluation, and Treatment of High Blood Pressure. National Heart, Lung, and Blood Institute, National Institutes of Health, May 2003; NIH publication no. 03-5233.

7. Campbell NR, Abbott D, Bass M et al. Self-measurement of blood pressure: recommendation of the Canadian Coalition for High Blood Pressure Prevention and Control. *Can J Cardiol.* 1995; 11(Suppl H):5H–17H.

Appendix 7-1.

Facts About Lowering Blood Pressure

High blood pressure is a serious condition, which often has no symptoms. Once high blood pressure occurs, it usually lasts a lifetime. But by taking action, you can prevent and control it.

This fact sheet will tell you what high blood pressure is, and how to prevent or control it.

What Is High Blood Pressure?

Blood pressure is the force of blood against the walls of arteries. Blood pressure rises and falls throughout the day. But when the pressure stays elevated over time, then it's called high blood pressure.

The medical term for high blood pressure is hypertension. High blood pressure is dangerous because it makes the heart work too hard and contributes to atherosclerosis (hardening of the arteries). It increases the risk of heart disease (see Box 1) and stroke, the first- and third-leading causes of death among Americans. High blood pressure also can result in other conditions, such as congestive heart failure, kidney disease, and blindness.

High blood pressure affects about 50 million—or one in four—American adults. Some people are

more likely to develop it than others. It is especially common among African Americans, who tend to develop it earlier and more often than whites. Also, many Americans tend to develop high blood pressure as they get older, but hypertension is *not* a part of healthy aging. About 60 percent of all Americans age 60 and older have high blood pressure.

Others at high risk of developing hypertension are the overweight, those with a family history of high blood pressure, and those with a high-normal blood pressure (see Box 2). High blood pressure also is more common in the southeastern United States.

How Is Blood Pressure Checked?

Blood pressure usually is measured in millimeters of mercury (mm Hg) and recorded as two numbers—systolic pressure (as the heart beats) "over" diastolic pressure (as the heart relaxes between beats)—for example, 130/80 mm Hg. Both numbers are important, although for some Americans systolic blood pressure is especially important (see Box 3).

The test to measure blood pressure is simple, quick, and painless. Typically, a blood pressure cuff called a sphygmomanometer (pronounced sfig'-mo-ma-nom-e-ter) is used. The cuff is placed around the upper arm and inflated with air until blood flow stops. Then, the cuff is slowly deflated, letting blood flow start again.

As the cuff is deflated, a stethoscope is used to listen to the blood flow in an artery at the inner elbow. The first thumping sound heard gives the blood pressure as the heart contracts—this is the systolic pressure. When the thumping sound is no longer heard, the blood pressure is between heartbeats—this is the diastolic pressure.

Because blood pressure changes and is affected by many factors, the test will be repeated on different days to confirm a reading of high blood pressure.

A systolic blood pressure of less than 120 and a diastolic blood pressure of less than 80 mm Hg are optimal. Systolic blood pressure of 140 or higher, or diastolic blood pressures of 90 or higher mm Hg are high. If systolic and diastolic pressures fall into different categories, go by the higher category. Even levels slightly above optimal can increase the risk of heart disease and other problems.

Box 1.
Risk Factors for Heart Disease

Risk factors are conditions or behaviors that increase your likelihood of developing a disease. When you have more than one for heart disease, your risk greatly multiplies. So if you have high blood pressure, you need to take action. Fortunately, most of the heart disease risk factors are largely within your control.

Risk factors under your control are:

- High blood pressure
- High blood cholesterol
- Cigarette smoking
- Diabetes
- Overweight
- Physical inactivity

Risk factors beyond your control are:

- Age (45 or older for men; 55 or older for women)
- Family history of early heart disease (having a mother or sister who has been diagnosed with heart disease before age 65, or a father or brother diagnosed before age 55)

Box 2.
Blood Pressure Levels for Adults[a]

Category	Systolic[b] (mmHg)[c]		Diastolic[b] (mmHg)[c]	Result
Optimal	less than 120	*and*	less than 80	Good for you!
Normal	less than 130	*and*	less than 85	Keep an eye on it.
High-Normal	130–139	*or*	85–89	Your blood pressure could be a problem. Make needed changes in what you eat and drink, get physical activity, and lose extra weight. If you also have diabetes, see the doctor.
Hypertension				All stages—You have high blood pressure.
Stage 1	140–159	*or*	90–99	
Stage 2	160–179	*or*	100–109	Ask your doctor or nurse how to control it.
Stage 3	180 or higher	*or*	110 or higher	

[a]For adults 18 and older who are not on medicine for high blood pressure and do not have a short-term serious illness. Source: The Sixth Report of the Joint National Committee on Prevention, Detection, Evaluation, and Treatment of High Blood Pressure, National High Blood Pressure Education Program, November 1997.

[b]If systolic and diastolic pressures fall into different categories, overall status is the higher category.

[c]Millimeters of mercury.

How Can You Prevent or Control High Blood Pressure?

Everyone can take steps to prevent high blood pressure or, for those who already have it, to keep it under control. The steps are:

- Maintain a healthy weight.
- Be physically active.
- Follow a healthy eating plan, which includes foods lower in salt and sodium.
- If you drink alcoholic beverages, do so in moderation.
- If you have high blood pressure and are prescribed medication, take it as directed.

Each of these steps is discussed more fully.

Maintain a Healthy Weight

Overweight increases your risk of developing high blood pressure. In fact, blood pressure rises as body weight increases. Losing even 10 pounds can lower blood pressure—and it has the biggest effect in those who are overweight and already have hypertension.

Overweight also is a risk factor for heart disease. And it increases your chance of developing high blood cholesterol and diabetes—two more risk factors for heart disease.

Box 3.
Watch That Systolic

Both numbers in a blood pressure test are important but, for some, the systolic is especially meaningful. That's because, for those middle aged and older, the systolic pressure gives the most accurate diagnosis of high blood pressure.

Systolic blood pressure is the top number in a blood pressure reading (see page 97). It is high if it is 140 mm Hg or above.

For American adults, the systolic pressure increases sharply with age, while the diastolic increases until about age 55 and then declines. Thus, many older Americans have only a high systolic pressure—a condition known as "isolated systolic hypertension," or ISH.

A high systolic pressure causes blood vessels to stiffen and can lead to cardiovascular disease and damage kidneys and other organs.

Clinical studies have proven that treating a high systolic pressure saves lives and greatly reduces illness. Yet, most Americans do not have their high systolic pressure under control.

Blood pressure must be controlled to under 140/90 mm Hg. The treatment is the same for ISH as for other forms of high blood pressure. So talk with your doctor. Ask about your blood pressure level—and especially your systolic blood pressure. If your blood pressure is too high, ask about adjusting your drug and making lifestyle changes to bring it to less than 140/90 mm Hg.

Box 4.
Calculate Your BMI

The formula for calculating BMI is:

$$BMI = \frac{\text{your weight in pounds}^*}{(\text{your height in inches})^2} \times 703$$

Or, try this simple 3-step method:

1) Multiply your weight in pounds* by 703
2) Divide the answer by your height (in inches)
3) Divide the answer again by your height (in inches) to get your BMI

For example: If you are 5′ 7″ tall (or 67″) and weigh 170 pounds, you would:

$170 \times 703 = 119,510$

$119,510/67 = 1,785$

$1,785/67 = 26.6$

BMI = 26.6
This BMI falls in the overweight category.

*Weight is measured with underwear but no shoes.

Two key measures are used to determine if someone is overweight. These are the body mass index, or BMI, and waist circumference.

BMI relates weight to height. It gives an approximation of total body fat—and that's what increases the risk of obesity-related diseases.

To find your BMI, use the formula in **Box 4**, or check the chart in **Box 5** for an approximate value. **Box 6** gives the BMI categories for men and women. Overweight is defined as a BMI of 25 to 29.9; obesity is defined as a BMI equal to or more than 30.

But BMI alone does not determine risk. For example, in someone who is very muscular or who has swelling from fluid retention (called edema), the BMI may overestimate body fat. BMI also may not accurately estimate total body fat in older persons or those losing muscle.

That's why waist measurement is often checked as well. Another reason is that too much body fat in the abdomen (or stomach area) also increases disease risk. A waist measurement of more than 35 inches in women and more than 40 inches in men is considered high.

The Box on page 100 offers guidelines on how to interpret BMI and waist measurements. It tells if you are at increased risk for disease and if you need to lose weight. If you fall in the obese range, you should lose weight. You also should lose weight if you are overweight or have a high waist measurement and two or more heart disease risk factors (**see Box 1**). If you fall in the normal weight range or are overweight but do need to lose pounds, you still should be careful not to gain weight.

If you have to lose weight, it's important to do so slowly. Lose no more than 1/2 to 2 pounds a week. Begin with a goal of losing 10 percent of your current weight. This is the healthiest way to lose weight and—importantly—it offers the best chance of long-term success.

There's no magic formula for weight loss. You have to eat fewer calories than you burn. Just how many calories you burn daily depends on factors such as your body size and how physically active you are (**see Box 7**).

One pound equals 3,500 calories. So, to lose 1 pound a week, you would need to eat 500 calories a day less or burn 500 calories a day more than you usually do. It's best to work out some combination of both eating less and being more physically active.

And remember to be careful of serving sizes. It's not only what you eat that adds calories, but also how much.

As you lose, be sure to eat a healthy diet, with a variety of foods. A good plan to follow is the one given on page 104. **Box 15** offers some tips to make the plan lower in calories.

Be Physically Active

Being physically active is one of the most important steps you can take to prevent or control high blood pressure. It also helps to reduce your risk of heart disease.

It doesn't take a lot of effort to become physically active. All you need to do is 30 minutes of moderate-level activity on most, and preferably all, days of the week. Examples of moderate level ac-

Box 5.
Body Mass Index

Here is a chart for men and women that gives the body mass index (BMI) for various heights and weights.*

	21	22	23	24	25	26	27	28	29	30	31
4'10"	100	105	110	115	119	124	129	134	138	143	148
5'0"	107	112	118	123	128	133	138	143	148	153	158
5'1"	111	116	122	127	132	137	143	148	153	158	164
5'3"	118	124	130	135	141	146	152	158	163	169	175
5'5"	126	132	138	144	150	156	162	168	174	180	186
5'7"	134	140	146	153	159	166	172	178	185	191	198
5'9"	142	149	155	162	169	176	182	189	196	203	209
6'.0"	150	157	165	172	179	186	193	200	208	215	222
6'1"	159	166	174	182	189	197	204	212	219	227	235
6'3"	168	176	184	192	200	208	216	224	232	240	248

* Weight is measured with underwear but no shoes.

Box 6.
What Does Your BMI Mean?

Category	BMI	Result
Normal weight	18.5–24.9	Good for you! Try not to gain weight.
Overweight	25–29.9	Do not gain any weight, especially if your waist measurement is high. You need to lose weight if you have two or more risk factors for heart disease (see page 97) and: • Are overweight, or • Have a high waist measurement.
Obese	30 or greater	You need to lose weight. Lose weight slowly—about 1/2–2 pounds a week. See your doctor or a nutritionist if you need help.

Source: *Clinical Guidelines on the Identification, Evaluation, and Treatment of Overweight and Obesity in Adults*, National Heart, Lung, and Blood Institute, in cooperation with the National Institute of Diabetes and Digestive and Kidney Diseases, National Institutes of Health, June 1998.

tivity are brisk walking, bicycling, raking leaves, and gardening. For more examples, see **Box 7**.

You can even divide the 30 minutes into shorter periods of at least 10 minutes each. For instance: Use stairs instead of an elevator; get off a bus one

Box 7.
Be Physically Active

Engage in at least 30 minutes of moderate-level activity on most, and preferably all, days of the week. Examples of moderate-level activity are:

- Walking briskly (3–4 miles per hour)
- Conditioning or general calisthenics
- Home care and general cleaning
- Home repair, such as painting
- Mowing the lawn (with power mower)
- Gardening
- Dancing
- Racket sports, such as table tennis
- Golf (walking the course)
- Fishing (standing and casting, walking, or wading)
- Swimming (with moderate effort)
- Cycling (at a moderate speed of 10 miles per hour or less)
- Canoeing or rowing (at a speed of about 2–3.9 miles per hour)

Source: Adapted from Pate, et al., *Journal of the American Medical Association*, 1995, Vol. 273, page 404.

or two stops early; or park your car at the far end of the lot at work. If you already engage in 30 minutes a day, you can get added benefits by doing more. Do a moderate-level activity for a longer period each day or engage in a more vigorous activity.

Most people don't need to see a doctor before they start a moderate-level physical activity. You should check first with a doctor if you have heart trouble or have had a heart attack, if you are over age 50 and are not used to doing a moderate-level activity, if you have a family history of heart disease at an early age, or if you have any other serious health problem.

To help get you started, a sample walking program is given on page 107.

Follow a Healthy Eating Plan, which Includes Foods Lower in Salt and Sodium

Research has shown that what you eat affects the development of high blood pressure. A healthy eating plan can both reduce the risk of developing high blood pressure and lower an already elevated blood pressure.

A key ingredient of healthy eating is choosing foods lower in salt (sodium chloride) and other forms of sodium. A recent study showed just how important lowering sodium is in keeping blood pressure at a healthy level (see **Box 19** on page 106).

Most Americans eat more salt and sodium than they need. Some people, such as African Americans and the elderly, are especially sensitive to salt and sodium and may need to be particularly careful about how much they consume.

Most Americans should consume no more than 2.4 grams (2,400 milligrams) of sodium a day. That equals 6 grams (about 1 teaspoon) of table salt a day. For someone with high blood pressure, the doctor may advise less.

The 6 grams includes ALL salt and sodium consumed, including that used in cooking and at the table. **Boxes 8** and **9** offer tips on how to choose and prepare foods lower in salt and sodium.

Sodium is found naturally in many foods. *But processed foods account for most of the salt and sodium Americans consume.* Processed foods with high amounts of salt include regular canned vegetables and soups, frozen dinners, lunch meats, instant and ready-to-eat cereals, and salty chips and other snacks. You should use food labels to choose products lower in sodium. **Boxes 10, 11,** and **12** can help you learn how to read and compare food labels.

Sodium also is found in many foods that may surprise you, such as baking soda, soy sauce, monosodium glutamate (MSG), seasoned salts, and some antacids—the range is wide.

Before trying salt substitutes, you should check with your doctor, especially if you have high blood pressure. These contain potassium chloride and may be harmful for those with certain medical conditions.

Box 8.
Tips to Reduce Salt and Sodium

- Buy fresh, plain frozen, or canned "with no salt added" vegetables.
- Use fresh poultry, fish, and lean meat, rather than canned or processed types.
- Use herbs, spices, and salt-free seasoning blends in cooking and at the table—**see Box 9** on ways to spice up food.
- Cook rice, pasta, and hot cereals without salt. Cut back on instant or flavored rice, pasta, and cereal mixes, which usually have added salt.
- Choose "convenience" foods that are lower in sodium. Cut back on frozen dinners, mixed dishes such as pizza, packaged mixes, canned soups or broths, and salad dressings—these often have a lot of sodium.
- Rinse canned foods, such as tuna, to remove some sodium.
- When available, buy low- or reduced-sodium, or no-salt-added versions of foods—**see Boxes 10, 11,** and **12** on how to use food labels for guidance.
- Choose ready-to-eat breakfast cereals that are lower in sodium.

For an overall eating plan, consider the DASH diet. DASH stands for "Dietary Approaches to Stop Hypertension." DASH was a clinical study that tested the effects on blood pressure of nutrients as they occur together in food. It found that blood pressures were reduced by an eating plan low in saturated fat, total fat, and cholesterol, and rich in fruits, vegetables, and lowfat dairy foods. The DASH diet includes whole grains, poultry, fish, and nuts, and has reduced amounts of fats, red meats, sweets, and sugared beverages. It also is rich in potassium, calcium, and magnesium, as well as protein and fiber.

A second study, called DASH-Sodium, found that even when using the DASH diet, lowering salt and sodium is important—blood pressure was lowest when both lifestyles were followed. See **Box 19** for more on the findings from DASH-Sodium about the effects of lowering salt.

Box 13 gives the servings and food groups for the DASH diet. The number of servings you require may vary, depending on your caloric need.

You should be aware that the DASH diet has more daily servings of fruits, vegetables, and grains than you may be used to eating. The servings make it high in fiber, which may temporarily cause bloating and diarrhea. To get used to the DASH diet, gradually increase your servings of fruits, veg-

Box 9.
Spice It Up

Make foods tasty without using salt. Try these flavorings, spices, and herbs:

For Meat, Poultry, and Fish—

Beef . . . . Bay leaf, marjoram, nutmeg, onion, pepper, sage, thyme

Lamb . . . . Curry powder, garlic, rosemary, mint

Pork . . . . Garlic, onion, sage, pepper, oregano

Veal . . . . Bay leaf, curry powder, ginger, marjoram, oregano

Chicken . . . . Ginger, marjoram, oregano, paprika, poultry seasoning, rosemary, sage, tarragon, thyme

Fish . . . . Curry powder, dill, dry mustard, lemon juice, marjoram, paprika, pepper

For Vegetables—

Carrots . . . . Cinnamon, cloves, marjoram, nutmeg, rosemary, sage

Corn . . . . Cumin, curry powder, onion, paprika, parsley

Green beans . . . . . . Dill, curry powder, lemon juice, marjoram, oregano, tarragon, thyme

Greens . . . . Onion, pepper

Peas . . . . Ginger, marjoram, onion, parsley, sage

Potatoes . . . . Dill, garlic, onion, paprika, parsley, sage

Summer squash . . . Cloves, curry powder, marjoram, nutmeg, rosemary, sage

Winter squash . . . . . Cinnamon, ginger, nutmeg, onion

Tomatoes . . . . Basil, bay leaf, dill, marjoram, onion, oregano, parsley, pepper

Box 10.
Label Language

Food labels can help you choose items lower in sodium. Look for labels on cans, boxes, bottles, bags, and other products that say:

- Sodium free
- Very low sodium
- Low sodium
- Light in sodium
- Reduced or less sodium
- Unsalted or no salt added

etables, and grains. **Box 18** offers some tips on how to adopt the DASH diet.

A good way to change to the DASH diet is to keep a diary of your current eating habits. Write down what you eat, how much, when, and why. Note whether or not you snack on high fat foods while watching television, or if you skip breakfast and eat a big lunch. Do this for several days. You'll be able to see where you can start making changes.

If you are trying to lose weight, you should choose an eating plan lower in calories. You can still use the DASH diet, but follow it at a lower calorie level (see **Box 14**). Again, a food diary can be helpful. It can tell you if there are certain times you eat but aren't really hungry, or when you can substitute lower-calorie foods for higher-calorie items.

If You Drink Alcoholic Beverages, Do So in Moderation

Drinking too much alcohol can raise blood pressure. It also can harm the liver, brain, and heart. Furthermore, alcoholic drinks contain calories, which matter if you are trying to lose weight.

If you drink alcoholic beverages, have only a moderate amount—one drink a day for women; two drinks a day for men.

What counts as a drink?

- 12 ounces of beer (regular or light, 150 calories),
- 5 ounces of wine (100 calories), or
- 1 1/2 ounces of 80-proof whiskey (100 calories)

If You Have High Blood Pressure and Are Prescribed Medication, Take It As Directed

If you have high blood pressure, the lifestyle habits noted above may not lower your blood pressure enough. If they don't, you will need to take medication.

Box 11.
Use the Food Label

Frozen Peas:

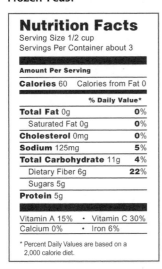

Nutrition Facts
Serving Size 1/2 cup
Servings Per Container about 3

Amount Per Serving	
Calories 60 Calories from Fat 0	
	% Daily Value*
Total Fat 0g	**0**%
Saturated Fat 0g	**0**%
Cholesterol 0mg	**0**%
Sodium 125mg	**5**%
Total Carbohydrate 11g	**4**%
Dietary Fiber 6g	**22**%
Sugars 5g	
Protein 5g	

Vitamin A 15%	•	Vitamin C 30%
Calcium 0%	•	Iron 6%

* Percent Daily Values are based on a 2,000 calorie diet.

Food labels can help you choose foods lower in sodium, as well as calories, saturated fat, total fat, and cholesterol. The label tells you:

Amount per Serving: Nutrient amounts are given for one serving. If you eat more or less than a serving, add or subtract amounts. For example, if you eat 1 cup of peas, you need to double the nutrient amounts on the label.

Nutrients: You'll find the milligrams of sodium in one serving.

Number of Servings: The serving size is 1/2 cup. The package contains about 3 servings.

Percent Daily Value: Percent Daily Value helps you compare products and tells you if the food is high or low in sodium. Choose products with the lowest Percent Daily Value for sodium.

Box 12.
Compare Labels

Which of these two items is lower in sodium? To tell, check the Percent Daily Value.

The answer is given below.

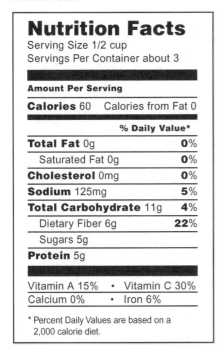

Frozen Peas:

Nutrition Facts
Serving Size 1/2 cup
Servings Per Container about 3

Amount Per Serving	
Calories 60 Calories from Fat 0	
	% Daily Value*
Total Fat 0g	**0**%
Saturated Fat 0g	**0**%
Cholesterol 0mg	**0**%
Sodium 125mg	**5**%
Total Carbohydrate 11g	**4**%
Dietary Fiber 6g	**22**%
Sugars 5g	
Protein 5g	

Vitamin A 15%	•	Vitamin C 30%
Calcium 0%	•	Iron 6%

* Percent Daily Values are based on a 2,000 calorie diet.

Canned Peas:

Nutrition Facts
Serving Size 1/2 cup
Servings Per Container about 3

Amount Per Serving	
Calories 60 Calories from Fat 0	
	% Daily Value*
Total Fat 0g	**0**%
Saturated Fat 0g	**0**%
Cholesterol 0mg	**0**%
Sodium 380mg	**16**%
Total Carbohydrate 12g	**4**%
Dietary Fiber 3g	**14**%
Sugars 4g	
Protein 4g	

Vitamin A 6%	•	Vitamin C 10%
Calcium 2%	•	Iron 8%

* Percent Daily Values are based on a 2,000 calorie diet.

ANSWER: The frozen peas. The canned peas have three times more sodium than the frozen peas.

Box 13.
The DASH Eating Plan

The DASH plan shown below is based on **2,000 calories a day**. The number of daily servings in a food group may vary from those listed depending on your caloric needs. (See Box 14 for more.)

Food Group	Daily Servings (except as noted)	Serving Sizes
Grains & grain products	7–8	1 slice bread
		1 cup ready-to-eat cereal*
		1/2 cup cooked rice, pasta, or cereal
Vegetables	4–5	1 cup raw leafy vegetable
		1/2 cup cooked vegetable
		6 ounces vegetable juice
Fruits	4–5	1 medium fruit
		1/4 cup dried fruit
		1/2 cup fresh, frozen, or canned fruit
		6 ounces fruit juice
Lowfat or fat free dairy foods	2–3	8 ounces milk
		1 cup yogurt
		1 1/2 ounces cheese
Lean meats, poultry, and fish	2 or less	3 ounces cooked lean meats, skinless poultry, or fish
Nuts, seeds, and dry beans	4–5 per week	1/3 cup or 1 1/2 ounces nuts
		1 tablespoon or 1/2 ounce seeds
		1/2 cup cooked dry beans
Fats & oils**	2–3	1 teaspoon soft margarine
		1 tablespoon lowfat mayonnaise
		2 tablespoons light salad dressing
		1 teaspoon vegetable oil
Sweets	5 per week	1 tablespoon sugar
		1 tablespoon jelly or jam
		1/2 ounce jelly beans
		8 ounces lemonade

*Serving sizes vary between 1/2-1 1/4 cups. Check the product's nutrition label.

**Fat content changes serving counts for fats and oils: For example, 1 tablespoon of regular salad dressing equals 1 serving; 1 tablespoon of a lowfat dressing equals 1/2 serving; 1 tablespoon of a fat free dressing equals 0 servings.

However, even if you do need medication, you still must follow the lifestyle changes. Doing so will help your medication work better and may reduce how much of it you need.

There are many drugs available to lower high blood pressure. They work in various ways. *Often, two or more drugs work better than one.*

Here's a rundown on the main types of drugs and how they work:

Diuretics—These are sometimes called "water pills" because they work in the kidney and flush excess water and sodium from the body through urine. This reduces the amount of fluid in the blood. And, since sodium is flushed out of blood vessel walls, the vessels open wider. Pressure goes down. There are different types of diuretics. They are often used with other high blood pressure drugs.

Beta-blockers—These reduce nerve impulses to the heart and blood vessels. This makes the heart beat less often and with less force. Blood pressure drops and the heart works less hard.

Angiotensin converting enzyme (ACE) inhibitors—These prevent the formation of a hormone called angiotensin II, which normally causes ves-

Box 14.
DASH Diet Servings for Other Calorie Levels

Food Group	Servings/Day at 1,600 calories/day	Servings/Day at 3,100 calories/day
Grains & grain products	6	12–13
Vegetables	3–4	6
Fruits	4	6
Lowfat or fat free dairy foods	2–3	3–4
Meats, poultry, and fish	1–2	2–3
Nuts, seeds, and dry beans	3/week	1
Fat & oils	2	4
Sweets	0	2

Box 15.
How to Lower Calories on the DASH Eating Plan

The DASH eating plan was not designed to promote weight loss. But it is rich in lower calorie foods, such as fruits and vegetables. You can make it lower in calories by replacing higher-calorie foods with more fruits and vegetables—and that also will make it easier for you to reach your DASH diet goals. Here are some examples:

To increase fruits—

- Eat a medium apple instead of four shortbread cookies. You'll save 80 calories.
- Eat 1/4 cup of dried apricots instead of a 2-ounce bag of pork rinds. You'll save 230 calories.

To increase vegetables—

- Have a hamburger that's 3 ounces instead of 6 ounces. Add a 1/2 cup serving of carrots and a 1/2 cup serving of spinach. You'll save more than 200 calories.
- Instead of 5 ounces of chicken, have a stir fry with 2 ounces of chicken and 1 1/2 cups of raw vegetables. Use a small amount of vegetable oil. You'll save 50 calories.

To increase lowfat or fat free dairy products—

- Have a 1/2 cup serving of lowfat frozen yogurt instead of a 1 1/2-ounce milk chocolate bar. You'll save about 110 calories.

And don't forget these calorie-saving tips:

- Use lowfat or fat free condiments, such as fat free salad dressings.
- Eat smaller portions—cut back gradually.
- Choose lowfat or fat free dairy products to reduce total fat intake.
- Use food labels to compare fat content in packaged foods. Items marked lowfat or fat free are not always lower in calories than their regular versions. See Boxes 11 and 12 on how to read and compare food labels.
- Limit foods with lots of added sugar, such as pies, flavored yogurts, candy bars, ice cream, sherbet, regular soft drinks, and fruit drinks.
- Eat fruits canned in their own juice.
- Add fruit to plain yogurt.
- Snack on fruit, vegetable sticks, unbuttered and unsalted popcorn, or bread sticks.
- Drink water or club soda.

sels to narrow. The blood vessels relax and pressure goes down.

Angiotensin antagonists—These are a new type of high blood pressure drug. They shield blood vessels from angiotensin II. As a result, the vessels are wider and pressure lowers.

Calcium channel blockers (CCBs)—These keep calcium from entering the muscle cells of the heart and blood vessels. Blood vessels relax and pressure goes down.

One short-acting type of CCB has been found to increase the chance of having another heart attack. Shortacting CCBs are taken several times a day. If you are on such a drug, you should talk with your doctor about other medication choices.

The finding does not apply to the longer-acting types of CCB, which are taken once a day.

Alpha blockers—These reduce nerve impulses to blood vessels, which allows blood to pass more easily.

Results from a clinical study indicate that an alpha blocker may not be the best choice for an initial treatment for high blood pressure. If you now take an alpha blocker drug for high blood pressure, consult with your doctor about whether or not your treatment should be modified.

Alpha-beta blockers—These work the same way as alpha blockers but also slow the heartbeat, as betablockers do. As a result, less blood is pumped through the vessels.

Nervous system inhibitors—These relax blood vessels by controlling nerve impulses.

Vasodilators—These directly open blood vessels by relaxing the muscle in the vessel walls.

When you start on a medication, work with your doctor to get the right drug and dose level for you. If you have side effects, tell your doctor so the medication can be adjusted. If you're worried about cost,

Box 16.
Get Those Nutrients

The DASH eating plan is rich in various nutrients believed to benefit blood pressure and in other factors involved in good health. The amounts of the nutrients vary by how much you eat. If you eat about 2,000 calories a day on the plan, the nutrients you will get include:

4,700	milligrams of potassium
500	milligrams of magnesium
1,240	milligrams of calcium
90	grams of protein
30	grams of fiber

Box 17.
Good Sources for Good Nutrients

Where's the potassium, calcium, and magnesium? Read on. (In the dairy products mentioned below, remember to choose lowfat or fat free types.)

Potassium—

catfish

lean pork

lean veal

cod

flounder

trout

milk

yogurt

dry peas and beans

green beans

apricots

peaches

bananas

prunes and prune juice

orange juice

lima beans

stewed tomatoes

spinach

plantain

sweet potatoes

pumpkin

potatoes

winter squash

Calcium—

cheese

milk

yogurt

tofu (made with calcium sulfate)

broccoli

spinach

turnip greens

mackerel

perch

salmon

Magnesium—

whole wheat bread

whole grain ready-to-eat and cooked cereals

broccoli

chard

spinach

okra

plantain

oysters

scallops

croaker

mackerel

sea bass

beans

soy milk

tofu

nuts and seeds

Box 18.
Tips on Making the Switch to the DASH Eating Plan

- Change gradually. Add a vegetable or fruit serving at lunch and dinner.

- Use only half the butter or margarine you do now.

- If you have trouble digesting dairy products, try lactase enzyme pills or drops—they're available at drugstores and groceries. Or buy lactose-free milk or milk with lactase enzyme added to it.

- Get added nutrients such as the B vitamins by choosing whole grain foods, including whole wheat bread or whole grain cereals.

- Spread out the servings. Have two servings of fruits and/ or vegetables at each meal, or add fruits as snacks.

- Treat meat as one part of the meal, instead of the focus. Try casseroles, pasta, and stir-fry dishes. Have two or more meatless meals a week.

- Use fruits or lowfat foods as desserts and snacks.

Box 19.
Lower Salt to Lower Blood Pressure

The DASH study occurred in two parts. DASH, the initial study, found that the eating plan given on page 104 reduced blood pressure. DASH-Sodium then examined the relationships between blood pressure, eating patterns, and various sodium intakes.

DASH-Sodium looked at the effect on blood pressure of three sodium levels: a "higher" intake of 3,200 milligrams per day (mg/day), which is similar to how much most Americans now consume, an "intermediate" intake of 2,400 mg/day, which is similar to the upper limit of current recommendations; and a "lower" intake of 1,400 mg/day.

The effect of each sodium level was tested for two diet plans: A "control" diet, typical of what many Americans eat, and the DASH diet.

Here are some key results:

- The less sodium consumed, the lower the blood pressure.

- Blood pressure was lower in the DASH diet than in the control diet at all three sodium levels.

- The lowest blood pressures occurred with the DASH diet at the lower sodium level.

- Sodium level had a bigger effect in the control diet than in the DASH diet.

- The effects of sodium reduction were seen in all study participants—those with and without high blood pressure, men and women, and African Americans and others.

DASH-Sodium shows the importance of lowering sodium intake—whatever your eating plan. But for a true winning combination, follow the DASH diet *and* lower your intake of salt.

tell your doctor or pharmacist—there may be a less expensive drug or a generic form that can be used instead.

It's important that you take the medication as prescribed, including in the right amount. That can prevent a heart attack, stroke, and congestive heart failure, a serious condition in which the heart cannot pump enough blood for the body's needs.

But you can be taking medication and still not have your blood pressure under control. Everyone—and older Americans in particular—must be careful to control their blood pressure to below 140/90 mm Hg. If your blood pressure is higher than that, talk with your doctor about adjusting your medication or making any needed lifestyle changes to bring your blood pressure down.

What Else Affects Blood Pressure?

Other factors have been reported to affect blood pressure. Here's a review of the latest findings:

- *Potassium.* Potassium helps to prevent and control blood pressure.
- *Calcium and Magnesium.* These nutrients may help prevent high blood pressure, and are important nutrients for other reasons too.

A note: The DASH eating plan is rich in potassium as well as calcium and magnesium. In fact, it has about two to three times the amounts that most Americans normally get in their diets—see **Box 16**.

You should try to get these nutrients from foods. So far, research on nutritional supplements has given inconclusive results. **Box 17** gives sources for each nutrient.

- *Fats.* Saturated fats and cholesterol in foods raise blood cholesterol, which increases the risk for heart disease. Foods high in fats also are high in calories, which must be reduced if you need to lose weight.
- *Caffeine.* This may cause blood pressure to rise but only temporarily. Unless you are sensitive

Box 20. A Sample Walking Program	Warm Up	Activity	Cool Down	Total Time
Week 1				
Session A	Walk slowly	Then walk briskly	Then walk slowly	
	5 min.	5 min.	5 min.	15 min.
Session B	Repeat above pattern			
Session C	Repeat above pattern			
Continue with at least three walking sessions during each week of the program.				
Week 2	Walk slowly	Walk briskly	Walk slowly	
	5 min.	7 min.	5 min.	17 min.
Week 3	Walk slowly	Walk briskly	Walk slowly	
	5 min.	9 min.	5 min.	19 min.
Week 4	Walk slowly	Walk briskly	Walk slowly	
	5 min.	11 min.	5 min.	21 min.
Week 5	Walk slowly	Walk briskly	Walk slowly	
	5 min.	13 min.	5 min.	23 min.
Week 6	Walk slowly	Walk briskly	Walk slowly	
	5 min.	15 min.	5 min.	25 min.
Week 7	Walk slowly	Walk briskly	Walk slowly	
	5 min.	18 min.	5 min.	28 min.
Week 8	Walk slowly	Walk briskly	Walk slowly	
	5 min.	20 min.	5 min.	30 min.
Week 9	Walk slowly	Walk briskly	Walk slowly	
	5 min.	23 min.	5 min.	33 min.
Week 10	Walk slowly	Walk briskly	Walk slowly	
	5 min.	26 min.	5 min.	36 min.
Week 11	Walk slowly	Walk briskly	Walk slowly	
	5 min.	28 min.	5 min.	38 min.
Week 12 and Beyond	Walk slowly	Walk briskly	Walk slowly	
	5 min.	30 min.	5 min.	40 min.

to caffeine, you do not have to limit how much you consume in order to prevent or control blood pressure.

- *Garlic or Onions.* These have not been found to affect blood pressure. But, they are tasty substitutes for salty seasonings and can be used often.
- *Stress Management.* Stress too can make blood pressure go up for a while, and it has been thought to contribute to high blood pressure. But the long-term effects of stress are as yet unclear. Furthermore, stress management techniques do not seem to prevent high blood

pressure. However, stress management techniques may help you control over-eating.

Here's a Recap

By preventing or controlling high blood pressure, you will reduce your risk for heart disease and stroke, as well as other conditions. The steps needed will help you feel healthier. Those steps are to:

- *Maintain a healthy weight.*
- *Be physically active.* It only takes 30 minutes of moderate-level physical activity on most, and preferably all, days of the week.
- *Follow a healthy eating plan, which includes foods lower in salt and sodium.* Have no more than 2,400 milligrams of sodium (6 grams of salt) a day. Also, try the DASH eating plan,

which is low in saturated fat, total fat, and cholesterol, and rich in fruits, vegetables, and lowfat dairy foods.

The DASH eating plan offers plenty of potassium, as well as calcium, magnesium, fiber, and protein.

- *If you drink alcoholic beverages, do so in moderation.*
- *If you have high blood pressure and are prescribed medication, take it as directed.*

Reprinted with permission from Facts About Lowering Blood Pressure, U.S Department of Health and Human Services, Public Health Service, National Institutes of Health, National Heart, Lung, and Blood Institute, NIH Publication No. 00-3281; Originally printed 1994; Reprinted October 1996; Revised May 2000.

Chapter 8:

Ongoing Evaluation and Management of the Ambulatory Patient with Hypertension

Tina M. Hisel and Jacqueline D. Joss

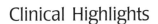

Clinical Highlights

Evaluating Response: Frequency of Clinic Visits

Assessing Progress toward Goals of Therapy

Modification of the Treatment Plan

- Considerations for Additional Therapy
- Inadequate Response to Therapy
- Resistant Hypertension

Patient Case

Key Points for Patients

References

Clinical Highlights

- How often should follow-up occur after initiating antihypertensive therapy?
- What type of evaluation should be performed during follow-up visits?
- What parameters should be taken into consideration when assessing the response to antihypertensive therapy?
- When is it necessary to add additional antihypertensive therapy?
- Which antihypertensive combinations are synergistic?

After initiating antihypertensive treatment, a periodic evaluation of the response to therapy will be necessary. Ongoing evaluation should occur at frequent intervals and include an assessment of blood pressure, risk factor and lifestyle modification, and target organ damage.

Evaluating Response: Frequency of Clinic Visits

The frequency of follow-up visits will depend on the level of blood pressure at baseline, the treatment options selected, and the cardiovascular risk status of the patient. The seventh report of the Joint National Committee on the Prevention, Detection, Evaluation, and Treatment of High Blood Pressure (JNC 7) has provided recommendations for follow-up after initiating antihypertensive therapy.[1] In general, it is recommended that follow-up occur at monthly intervals until the blood pressure goal is achieved.[1] Closer follow-up is necessary for patients with stage 2 hypertension, complicating comorbid conditions, and in patients exhibiting target organ damage.[1] Once blood pressure is stabilized, follow-up visits should be scheduled every 3–6 months.[1]

Another factor to take into consideration when determining follow-up is the time for pharmacologic therapies to achieve their optimal antihypertensive effect. It may take 2–4 weeks before the maximal blood-pressure-lowering effects are observed. Frequent monitoring will allow the clinician to titrate doses more rapidly in an effort to achieve individual blood pressure goals.

The frequency of follow-up should also be based on the need for laboratory tests. As discussed in Chapter 3, certain pharmacologic therapies such as angiotensin-converting enzyme (ACE) inhibitors, angiotensin II receptor blockers, and diuretics can adversely affect renal function and electrolytes. Therefore, treatment with these agents requires frequent laboratory follow-up. Although no specific recommendations are provided by pharmaceutical manufacturers, it is generally recommended to monitor serum creatinine and potassium 2 and 4 weeks after initiating therapy with an ACE inhibitor.[2] These laboratory parameters should be repeated 2 weeks after any dosage titration and every 3–6 months during stable maintenance therapy.[2] More frequent monitoring is necessary in patients at risk for hyperkalemia (preexisting renal impairment, diabetes, potassium-sparing diuretics, potassium supplements) or renal deterioration (preexisting renal impairment, congestive heart failure, diabetes, intensive diuretic therapy).[2]

Periodic evaluation of electrolytes, serum creatinine, and BUN (to evaluate for fluid contraction) should be conducted after initiating therapy with a thiazide or potassium-sparing diuretic. More frequent monitoring should occur in patients at risk for hyper/hypokalemia or renal deterioration.

Assessing Progress toward Goals of Therapy

As discussed in Chapter 4, goals of therapy should be established for all patients with hypertension, including blood pressure and cardiovascular risk factors (**Table 8-1**). Once treatments are initiated, a periodic assessment of the patient's progress toward these goals should be conducted. It is very important that blood pressure be monitored on an ongoing basis. Different methods for measuring blood pressure are available, including clinic, home, and ambulatory monitoring. Although all three methods have potential sources for error, valuable information can be obtained from each method.

Clinic measurement is the principle method for assessing blood pressure control. However, this method only provides an estimate of *average* blood pressure, tends to be higher than ambulatory measurements, and may be falsely elevated in patients with *white coat* hypertension.[5] Self-measurement by patients can serve as a useful adjunct to clinic measurements as it eliminates the white coat effect and allows for more frequent monitoring of blood pressure during normal everyday activities. In situations where there is a discrepancy between home and clinic measurements, further assessment is needed. The home monitor should be evaluated for accuracy and the correct technique for measuring blood pressure should be reviewed with the patient.

Noninvasive ambulatory blood pressure monitoring (ABPM) is an additional tool that can be used to evaluate blood pressure. Patients wear the ABPM device for 24 hours, which allows measurement of blood pressure at frequent intervals during daily activities and sleep (50–75 recordings over 24 hours).[6] The JNC 7 guidelines recommend the use of ABPM in several situations, including evaluation of patients with suspected white coat hypertension, episodic hypertension, and autonomic dysfunction.[1] It is also useful for evaluating drug resistance and hypotensive symptoms with antihypertensive therapy.[1] ABPM has been shown to be a better predictor for cardiovascular risk than clinic monitoring and can provide a more thorough assessment of overall blood pressure control.[7–9] Pharmacists are becoming increasingly involved with ABPM.[6,10]

In addition to reevaluating blood pressure, clinicians should continue to assess cardiovascular risk factors. It is critical that patients with comorbid conditions (e.g., hyperlipidemia, diabetes) are meeting their individual goals of therapy in an ef-

Table 8-1.
Goals of Therapy for Patients with Hypertension

Blood Pressure[1]		
Uncomplicated hypertension	<140/90 mm Hg	
Diabetes mellitus or chronic kidney disease	<130/80 mm Hg	
Dyslipidemia[3]	LDL, mg/dl	Non-HDL, mg/dl
Coronary heart disease (CHD) and CHD risk equivalents*(10-year risk for CHD >20%)	<100	<130
Multiple (2+) risk factors	<130	<160
0–1 risk factor	<160	<190
Diabetes Mellitus[4]		
Preprandial plasma glucose	90–130 mg/dl	
Peak postprandial plasma glucose	<180 mg/dl	
A1c	<7%	
Lifestyle Modifications		
Smoking cessation		
Physical activity		
Weight loss		
Limitation of alcohol, caffeine, salt, dietary fat, and cholesterol		

* CHD risk equivalents: peripheral arterial disease, abdominal aortic aneurysm, symptomatic carotid artery disease, diabetes, and multiple-risk factors conferring a 10-year risk for CHD >20%.

fort to reduce overall morbidity and mortality. Evaluation of lifestyle modifications, including smoking status, physical activity, weight reduction, and moderation of alcohol, caffeine, and sodium, should also be conducted. Periodic assessment of target organ damage should also occur. This includes obtaining an ECG or echocardiogram, performing fundoscopic examinations, and evaluation of serum creatinine, creatinine clearance, and urinary excretion of albumin.

Modification of the Treatment Plan

Considerations for Additional Therapy

If patients fail to achieve their blood pressure goal after the initial intervention, the treatment plan should be modified. One approach for those patients on monotherapy is to increase the dose of the antihypertensive medication to the maximally effective dose.[11] However, this may result in unwanted adverse effects for the patient, with little additional blood-pressure-lowering effects. It has been noted that most patients will require two or more antihypertensive medications to achieve their blood pressure goal.[1] An alternative approach is to use combination therapy. This has been associated with an 8–15% reduction in both systolic and diastolic blood pressure compared to 4–8% as seen with monotherapy.[12] As described in Chapter 6, this is the initial approach to treating patients whose blood pressure is greater than 20/10 mm Hg above their goal. When selecting combination therapy, two drugs with different mechanisms of action should be selected.[1] Several drug combinations have been shown to act synergistically to reduce blood pressure and some examples are given in **Table 8-2**. Some available proprietary combination products are listed in **Table 8-3**.

Inadequate Response to Therapy

Several factors have been shown to contribute to a lack of response to antihypertensive therapy (**Table 8-4**). Nonadherence has been recognized as a major contributing factor. The National Council on Patient Information and Education reported that up to 60% of all prescribed medications are taken incorrectly or not at all.[14] Nonadherence appears to affect all ages and socioeconomic classes. Even

Table 8-2.
Effective Antihypertensive Drug Combinations[13]

- Diuretic and beta-blocker
- Diuretic and ACE inhibitor
- Diuretic and angiotensin II receptor blocker
- Diuretic and calcium channel antagonist
- Calcium channel antagonist (dihydropyridine) and beta-blocker
- Calcium channel antagonist and ACE inhibitor
- Calcium channel antagonist and angiotensin II receptor blocker
- Alpha-blocker and beta-blocker

physicians themselves have been reported to take only 75% of prescribed medications correctly. Elderly patients are at higher risk for nonadherence, in part because of the quantity of medications they take.

As discussed in previous chapters, there are a number of factors that influence adherence (**Table 8-5**). Common causes of nonadherence include cost of medications, adverse effects, and complexity of the medication regimen. An assessment of the patient's ability to pay for medications should be conducted routinely. If cost is an issue, efforts should be made to prescribe generic medications. However, treatment with proprietary medications may be necessary. In this situation, clinicians can attempt to enroll patients in medication assistance programs that are available through many pharmaceutical manufacturers (e.g., rxassist.org, needymeds.com). Another option for reducing drug costs involves the splitting of tablets. **Table 8-6** depicts many products that can be split in half. It should be noted that splitting tablets may make a medication regimen more complex, and the resultant cost savings may be at the expense of adherence.

All antihypertensive treatments have the potential to cause unwanted adverse reactions (refer to Chapter 5 for specific drug-related adverse effects). Some pharmacologic agents have a favorable adverse event profile and are generally well tolerated (e.g., thiazide diuretics). However, other agents are associated with more severe adverse effects that can significantly impact a patient's quality of life (e.g., erectile dysfunction, fatigue with beta-blockers). An assessment of adverse effects should be conducted during every clinic visit and the treatment plan

Table 8-3.

Commercially Available Antihypertensive Drug Combinations[11,15]

Drug		Trade Name	Retail Cost Per Month*	Quantity
ACE Inhibitors				
Benazepril hydrochloride	*Hydrochlorothiazide*	*Lotensin HCT®*		
5 mg	6.25 mg		$31	30
10 mg	12.5 mg		$31	30
20 mg	12.5 mg		$31	30
20 mg	25 mg		$31	30
Captopril	*Hydrochlorothiazide*	*Generic*		
25 mg	15 mg		$33	60
25 mg	25 mg		$33	60
50 mg	15 mg		$54	60
50 mg	25 mg		$54	60
Enalapril maleate	*Hydrochlorothiazide*	*Generic*		
5 mg	12.5 mg		$24	30
10 mg	25 mg		N/A	
Fosinopril sodium	*Hydrochlorothiazide*	*Monopril-HCT®*		
10 mg	12.5 mg		$71	30
20 mg	25 mg		$71	30
Lisinopril	*Hydrochlorothiazide*	*Generic*		
10 mg	12.5 mg		$20	30
20 mg	12.5 mg		$22	30
20 mg	25 mg		$22	30
Moexipril hydrochloride	*Hydrochlorothiazide*	*Uniretic®*		
7.5 mg	12.5 mg		$30	30
15 mg	25 mg		$30	30
Quinapril hydrochloride	*Hydrochlorothiazide*	*Accuretic®*		
10 mg	12.5 mg		$32	30
20 mg	12.5 mg		$32	30
20 mg	25 mg		$32	30
Angiotensin II Receptor Blockers and Diuretics				
Candesartan cilexetil	*Hydrochlorothiazide*	*Atacand HCT®*		
16 mg	12.5 mg		$57	30
32 mg	12.5 mg		$57	30
Eprosartan mesylate	*Hydrochlorothiazide*	*Teveten HCT®*		
600 mg	12.5 mg		N/A	
600 mg	25 mg		N/A	
Irbesartan	*Hydrochlorothiazide*	*Avalide®*		
150 mg	12.5 mg		$54	30
300 mg	12.5 mg		$57	30
Losartan potassium	*Hydrochlorothiazide*	*Hyzaar®*		
50 mg	12.5 mg		$43	30
100 mg	25 mg		$59	30
Olmesartan medoxomil	*Hydrochlorothiazide*	*Benicar HCT®*		
20 mg	12.5 mg		N/A	

(continued)

Table 8-3. *(continued)*

Commercially Available Antihypertensive Drug Combinations[11,15]

Drug		Trade Name	Retail Cost Per Month*	Quantity
Angiotensin II Receptor Blockers and Diuretics				
Olmesartan medoxomil	*Hydrochlorothiazide*	*Benicar HCT®*		
40 mg	12.5 mg		$48	2
40 mg	25 mg		$48	2
Telmisartan	*Hydrochlorothiazide*	*Micardis HCT®*		
40 mg	12.5 mg		$41	30
80 mg	12.5 mg		$47	30
Valsartan	*Hydrochlorothiazide*	*Diovan HCT®*		
80 mg	12.5 mg		$48	30
160 mg	12.5 mg		$53	30
Beta-Blockers and Diuretics				
Atenolol	*Chlorthalidone*	*Generic*		
50 mg	25 mg		$11	30
100 mg	25 mg		$11	30
Bisoprolol fumarate	*Hydrochlorothiazide*	*Generic*		
2.5 mg	6.25 mg		$23	30
5 mg	6.25 mg		$23	30
10 mg	6.25 mg		$23	30
Metoprolol tartrate	*Hydrochlorothiazide*	*Lopressor HCT®*		
50 mg	25 mg		$58	60
100 mg	25 mg		$92	60
100 mg	50 mg		$48	30
Propranolol hydrochloride	*Hydrochlorothiazide*	*Generic*		
40 mg	25 mg		$11	60
80 mg	25 mg		$11	60
Propranolol hydrochloride extended release	*Hydrochlorothiazide*	*Inderide LA®*		
80 mg	50 mg		$54	30
120 mg	50 mg		$67	30
160 mg	50 mg		$75	30
Timolol maleate	*Hydrochlorothiazide*	*Timolide®*		
10 mg	25 mg		$48	60
Diuretic Combinations				
Hydrochlorothiazide	*Spironolactone*	*Generic*		
25 mg	25 mg		$10	30
50 mg	50 mg		N/A	
Hydrochlorothiazide	*Triamterene*	*Generic*		
25 mg	37.5 mg		$8	30
50 mg	75 mg		$8	30
Hydrochlorothiazide	*Amiloride Hydrochloride*	*Generic*		
50 mg	5 mg		$8	30

(continued)

Table 8-3. *(continued)*
Commercially Available Antihypertensive Drug Combinations[11,15]

Drug		Trade Name	Retail Cost Per Month*	Quantity
Direct Vasodilators and Diuretics				
Hydralazine hydrochloride	*Hydrochlorothiazide*	*Generic*		
25 mg	25 mg		$11	30
50 mg	50 mg		$15	30
100 mg	50 mg		$16	30
Central Alpha-Adrenergic Agonists and Diuretics				
Methyldopa	*Hydrochlorothiazide*	*Aldoril®*		
250 mg	15 mg		$34	60
250 mg	25 mg		$40	60
500 mg	30 mg		N/A	
500 mg	50 mg		$64	60
Clonidine hydrochloride	*Chlorthalidone*	*Generic*		
0.1 mg	15 mg		$55	60
0.2 mg	15 mg		$75	60
0.3 mg	15 mg		N/A	
Calcium Channel Antagonists and ACE Inhibitors				
Amlodipine besylate	*Benazepril*	*Lotrel®*		
2.5 mg	10 mg		$59	30
5 mg	10 mg		$59	30
5 mg	20 mg		$66	30
10 mg	20 mg		$72	30
Felodipine	*Enalapril maleate*	*Lexxel®*		
5 mg	2.5 mg		$48	30
5 mg	5 mg		$48	30
Verapamil hydrochloride	*Trandolapril*	*Tarka®*		
180 mg	2 mg		$57	30
240 mg	1 mg		$57	30
240 mg	2 mg		$57	30
240 mg	4 mg		$57	30

*Retail price obtained from www.drugstore.com (accessed October 2003). N/A = price not available.

should be modified if the current therapy adversely affects a patient's quality of life.

Nonadherence may be due to the complexity of the medication regimen. Patients with hypertension often have other comorbid conditions and may be taking numerous medications. Medication boxes and calendars (**Figure 8-1**) are available and may help simplify the medication regimen for individual patients. Once- and twice-daily dosing regimens are associated with better adherence than those that require more frequent administration. Many anti-hypertensive treatments are available in long-acting formulations which can be given once daily. Less frequent administration of medications may improve adherence and will likely improve quality of life. Additional recommendations to improve patient adherence are listed in **Table 8-7.**

Resistant Hypertension

Patients who fail to achieve their blood pressure goal despite treatment with three antihypertensive

Table 8-4.
Causes of Resistant Hypertension[1]

Volume Overload and Pseudotolerance

- Excess sodium intake
- Volume retention from kidney disease
- Inadequate diuretic therapy

Drug-Induced or Other Causes

- Nonadherence with antihypertensive medications
- Inadequate doses of antihypertensive medications
- Inappropriate combinations of antihypertensive medications
- Nonsteroidal anti-inflammatory drugs, cyclooxygenase 2 inhibitors
- Cocaine, amphetamines, other illicit drugs
- Sympathomimetics (decongestants, anorectics)
- Oral contraceptives
- Adrenal steroids
- Cyclosporine and tacrolimus
- Epoetin alfa (erythropoietin)
- Black licorice (including some chewing tobacco)
- Selected over-the-counter dietary supplements and medicines (e.g., ephedra, ma haung, bitter orange)

Associated Conditions

- Obesity
- Excess alcohol intake

Identifiable causes of hypertension as well as improper blood pressure measurement

Table 8-5.
Factors Influencing Medication Adherence[16]

Patient-Related Factors

- Age
- Educational background
- Socioeconomic status
- Employment status
- Ethnicity
- Cognitive impairment
- Lifestyle
- Physical impairment
- Absence of symptoms
- Understanding of hypertension and consequences
- Acceptance of the diagnosis
- Motivation of the patient and the family
- Adverse drug reactions
- Asymptomatic disease needing chronic therapy
- Belief that medication will not work
- Utilizing multiple pharmacies to fill prescriptions

Drug-Related Factors

- Number of doses per day
- Complexity of regimen
- Size and taste of tablets
- Packaging
- Cost of medication
- Difficult route of administration

Patient–Health Care Provider Relationship

- Access to health care provider
- Quality of the interaction
- Involvement of patient in decisions
- Attitude of health care provider toward patient and the treatment
- Quality of the communication and the information provided
- Interval between visits

medications (including a diuretic) are considered to have *resistant* hypertension.[1] Individuals with isolated systolic blood pressure are considered to have resistant hypertension if they are unable to reduce their systolic blood pressure to <160 mm Hg despite triple antihypertensive therapy.[11] Several factors have been identified that may contribute to resistant hypertension (**Table 8-4**), with volume overload being the most frequent cause.[11] Patients should be referred to a hypertension specialist if adequate blood pressure control cannot be achieved.

Table 8-6.
Comparison of Antihypertensive Treatments*

Drug	Dose	Tablet-Splitting	Retail Cost Per Month
ACE Inhibitors			
Benazepril (Lotensin®)		✂, not scored	
	5 mg QD		$31
	10 mg QD		$31
	20 mg QD		$31
	40 mg QD		$31
Captopril		✂, scored	
	12.5 mg tid		$10
	25 mg tid		$11
	50 mg tid		$10
	100 mg tid		$13
Enalapril		✂, not scored	
	2.5 mg bid		$11
	5 mg bid		$11
	10 mg bid		$22
	20 mg bid		$22
Fosinopril (Monopril®)		✂, not scored	
	10 mg QD		$33
	20 mg QD		$33
	40 mg QD		$33
Lisinopril		✂, not scored	
	2.5 mg QD		$13
	5 mg QD		$19
	10 mg QD		$19
	20 mg QD		$19
	40 mg QD		$24
Moexipril (Univasc®)		✂, scored	
	7.5 mg QD		$27
	15 mg QD		$27
Perindopril (Aceon®)		✂, not scored	
	2 mg QD		$32
	4 mg QD		$32
	8 mg QD		$49
Quinapril (Accupril®)		cannot be split	
	10 mg QD		$32
	20 mg QD		$32
	40 mg QD		$32
Ramipril (Altace®)		cannot be split	
	1.25 mg QD		$26
	2.5 mg QD		$34
	5 mg QD		$37
			$44

(continued)

Table 8-6. *(continued)*
Comparison of Antihypertensive Treatments*

Drug	Dose	Tablet-Splitting	Retail Cost Per Month
Trandolapril (Mavik®)		✂, not scored	
	1 mg		$30
	2 mg		$30
	4 mg		$30
Angiotensin II Receptor Blockers			
Candesartan (Atacand®)		✂, not scored	
	4 mg QD		$41
	8 mg QD		$41
	16 mg QD		$41
Eprosartan (Teveten®)		✂, scored	
	400 mg QD		$31
	600 mg QD		$41
Irbesartan (Avapro®)		✂, not scored	
	75 mg QD		$40
	150 mg QD		$45
	300 mg QD		$52
Losartan (Cozaar®)		cannot be split	
	25 mg QD		$43
	50 mg QD		$43
	100 mg QD		$58
Olmesartan (Benicar®)		✂, scored	
	20 mg QD		$37
	40 mg QD		$37
Telmisartan (Micardis®)		✂, scored	
	20 mg QD		$40
	40 mg QD		$40
	80 mg QD		$43
Valsartan (Diovan®)		cannot be split	
	80 mg QD		$43
	160 mg QD		$46
	320 mg QD		$58
Alpha-Blockers			
Doxazosin		✂, scored	
	1 mg QD		$20
	2 mg QD		$20
	4 mg QD		$22
	8 mg QD		$23
Prazosin		cannot be split	
	1 mg tid		$13
	2 mg tid		$17
			$25

(continued)

Table 8-6. *(continued)*
Comparison of Antihypertensive Treatments*

Drug	Dose	Tablet-Splitting	Retail Cost Per Month
Terazosin		cannot be split	
	1 mg QD		$14
	2 mg QD		$14
	5 mg QD		$14
	10 mg QD		$14
Beta-Blockers			
Atenolol		✂, scored	
	25 mg QD		$4
	50 mg QD		$4
	100 mg QD		$4
Labetalol		✂, scored	
	100 mg bid		$29
	200 mg bid		$40
	300 mg bid		$54
Metoprolol tartrate		✂, scored	
	50 mg bid		$10
	100 mg bid		$14
Metoprolol (Toprol XL®)		✂, scored	
	25 mg QD		$22
	50 mg QD		$22
	100 mg QD		$31
	200 mg QD		$59
Propranolol		cannot be split	
	10 mg bid		$5
	20 mg bid		$5
	40 mg bid		$8
	80 mg bid		$12
Propranolol extended release (Inderal® LA)		cannot be split	
	60 mg QD		$39
	80 mg QD		$42
	120 mg QD		$52
Calcium Channel Antagonists			
Amlodipine (Norvasc®)		✂, not scored	
	2.5 mg QD		$42
	5 mg QD		$42
	10 mg QD		$59
Diltiazem (Cardizem® CD)		cannot be split	
	120 mg QD		$41
	180 mg QD		$51
	240 mg QD		$70
	300 mg QD		$87
	360 mg QD		$95

(continued)

Table 8-6. *(continued)*
Comparison of Antihypertensive Treatments*

Drug	Dose	Tablet-Splitting	Retail Cost Per Month
Diltiazem (Tiazac®)		cannotbesplit	
	120 mg QD		$26
	180 mg QD		$34
	240 mg QD		$61
	300 mg QD		$77
	360 mg QD		$78
Felodipine (Plendil®)		cannot be split	
	2.5 mg QD		$35
	5 mg QD		$35
	10 mg QD		$60
Nifedipine extended release (Adalat® CC)		cannot be split	
	30 mg QD		$38
	60 mg QD		$67
	90 mg QD		$79
Verapamil extended release (Isoptin® SR)		✂, scored	
	120 mg QD		$36
	180 mg QD		$45
	240 mg QD		$50
Diuretics			
Hydrochlorothiazide		✂, scored	
	25 mg QD		$3
Chlorthalidone		✂, scored	
	25 mg QD		$8
	50 mg QD		$8
	100 mg QD		$8
Spironolactone		✂, scored	
	25 mg QD		$10
	50 mg QD		$20
	100 mg QD		$35
Hydrochlorothiazide/triamterene		✂, scored	
	25/37.5 mg		$18
	50/75 mg		$38

*✂ = scored, ✂, not scored = tablets can be split; however, the tablets are not scored.

Retail prices obtained from www.drugstore.com prices (accessed October 2003). Retail price reflects cost for 30 days' supply using full-sized tablets. Cost would be reduced by 50% if tablets were split.

Figure 8-1.
Example of a Medication Calendar

Medication	Before Breakfast	With Breakfast	Before Lunch	With Lunch	Before Dinner	With Dinner	Bedtime

Table 8-7.
General Guidelines to Improve Patient Adherence to Antihypertensive Therapy[11]

- Be aware of signs of patient nonadherence to antihypertensive therapy.
- Establish the goal of therapy: to reduce blood pressure to nonhypertensive levels with minimal or no adverse effects.
- Educate patients about the disease, and involve them and their families in its treatment. Have them measure blood pressure at home.
- Maintain contact with patients; consider telecommunication.
- Keep care inexpensive and simple.
- Encourage lifestyle modifications.
- Integrate medication regimen into routine activities of daily living.
- Prescribe medications according to pharmacologic principles, favoring long-acting formulations.
- Be willing to stop unsuccessful therapy and try a different approach.
- Anticipate adverse effects, and adjust therapy to prevent, minimize, or ameliorate side effects.
- Continue to add effective and tolerated drugs, stepwise, in sufficient doses to achieve the therapeutic goal.
- Encourage a positive attitude about achieving therapeutic goals.
- Consider using nurse case management.

Patient Case

1 PS is a 56-year-old male whose past medical history is significant for depression, obesity (BMI 31 kg/m^2), gastroesophageal reflux disease, and tobacco abuse. His current medications include sertraline 50 mg QD and omeprazole 20 mg QD. He was recently diagnosed with stage 1 hypertension after repeated blood pressure measurements demonstrated an average blood pressure of 155/90 mm Hg. He was subsequently started on hydrochlorothiazide 12.5 mg QD 1 month ago. He presents to clinic today for a follow-up visit. He states that he has been monitoring his blood pressure at home and reports that his systolic blood pressure has ranged from 140 to 150 mm Hg and his diastolic blood pressure has ranged from 70 to 80 mm Hg. His blood pressure during his clinic visit today was 145/80 mm Hg and it is noted that he has lost 5 pounds since his last visit. He does not report any adverse effects from hydrochlorothiazide and states that he has been adherent with this medication.

Question: **What would be your recommendation based on his blood pressure measurements at home and during his clinic visit today?**

Prior to recommending additional pharmacologic therapy, PS should be questioned about lifestyle modifications, including tobacco use, salt restriction, alcohol and caffeine use, and physical activity. He reports that he has stopped adding salt to his food and is restricting the amount of processed foods he is eating. He continues to smoke one pack of cigarettes per day and is interested in quitting. He only drinks alcohol occasionally and has switched to caffeine-free beverages. He has also started walking 30 minutes 4 days per week.

PS is complying well with lifestyle modifications, however he has not yet reached his blood pressure goal of <140/90 mm Hg. Since he is tolerating hydrochlorothiazide well and it is an inexpensive medication, it would seem reasonable to increase the dose to 25 mg daily. Another option would be to add a second drug with a different mechanism of action. As described in the JNC 7 guidelines, most patients with hypertension will require two or more antihypertensive medications to achieve their blood pressure goal. Smoking cessation options should also be discussed with PS as he is interested in quitting.

Question: **In addition to his blood pressure, what other type of evaluation should take place during his clinic visit today?**

Assessment for additional cardiovascular risk factors is essential. Measurement of a fasting glucose level and lipid panel should be performed if this has not been done previously. He should be encouraged to continue to lose weight in an effort to reduce his BMI to <25 kg/m^2. Potassium, serum creatinine, and BUN should also be monitored during his visit as he is currently receiving treatment with a diuretic.

Question: **When would you recommend that PS return for a clinic visit?**

Monthly follow-up visits are recommended until PS reaches his blood pressure goal. He should continue to monitor his blood pressure at home and a potassium, serum creatinine, and BUN should be measured at his next visit.

Key Points for Patients

- Once treatments are initiated for hypertension, frequent follow-up will be necessary until a patient's blood pressure is at goal.
- If blood pressure is not adequately controlled based on clinic measurements, a patient's health care provider may suggest monitoring blood pressure at home and reporting the measurements during follow-up visits.
- Many patients will require treatment with more than one blood pressure medication to adequately control blood pressure.
- Patients should notify their health care providers if it is difficult to take the prescribed medications for any reason.
- In an effort to minimize the number of medications taken, it is important for patients to modify their lifestyle, including salt, alcohol, and caffeine restriction; tobacco cessation; physical activity; and weight loss.

References

1. The seventh report of the Joint National Committee on Prevention, Detection, Evaluation, and Treatment of High Blood Pressure. The JNC 7 report. *JAMA*. 2003; 289:2560–71.

2. Micromedex® Healthcare Series: Micromedex, Greenwood Village, Colorado (edition expires 3/2004).

3. Expert Panel on Detection, Evaluation, and Treatment of High Blood Cholesterol in Adults. Executive summary of the third report of the National Cholesterol Education Program (NCEP) Expert Panel on Detection, Evaluation, and Treatment of High Blood Cholesterol in Adults (Adult Treatment Panel III). *JAMA*. 2001; 285:2486–97.

4. American Diabetes Association. Standards of medical care for patients with diabetes mellitus. *Diabetes Care*. 2003; 26:S33–50.

5. Pickering T. Principles and techniques of blood pressure measurement. *Cardiol Clin*. 2002; 20(2):207–23.

6. Ernst M, Bergus G. Noninvasive 24-hour ambulatory blood pressure monitoring: overview of technology and clinical applications. *Pharmacotherapy*. 2002; 22:597–612.

7. Perloff D, Sokolow M. Ambulatory blood pressure: mortality and morbidity. *J Hypertens Suppl*. 1991 Dec; 9(8):S31–3.

8. Perloff D, Sokolow M, Cowan R et al. Prognostic value of ambulatory blood pressure measurements: further analyses. *J Hypertens Suppl*. 1989 May; 7(3):S3–10.

9. Staessen J, Thijs L, Fagard R et al. Predicting cardiovascular risk using conventional vs ambulatory blood pressure in older patients with systolic hypertension. *JAMA*. 2000; 282:539–46.

10. Gardner S, Schneider E. 24-Hour ambulatory blood pressure monitoring in primary care. *J Am Board Fam Pract*. 2001; 14:166–71.

11. The sixth report of the Joint National Committee on Prevention, Detection, Evaluation, and Treatment of High Blood Pressure. *Arch Intern Med*. 1997; 157:2413–46.

12. Guidelines Subcommittee of the World Health Organization–International Society of Hypertension (WHO–ISH). 1999 World Health Organization–International Society of Hypertension guidelines for the management of hypertension. *J Hypertens*. 1999; 17:151–83.

13. Guidelines Committee of the European Society of Hypertension and European Society of Cardiology. 2003 European Society of Hypertension–European Society of Cardiology guidelines for the management of arterial hypertension. *J Hypertens*. 2003; 21:1011–53.

14. ScriptAssist Medication Compliance Programs. Noncompliance rates. http://www.scriptassistllc.com/noncomplianceRates.asp (accessed 2003 July 2).

15. Treatment guidelines from the *Medical Letter*. Drugs for hypertension. *Med. Lett*. 2003; 1(6):33–40.

16. Waeber B, Burnier M, Brunner H. How to improve adherence with prescribed treatment in hypertensive patients? *J Cardiovasc Pharmacol*. 2000; 35(S3): S23–6.

Chapter 9:

Referral to Other Health Care Providers

Alan H. Mutnick

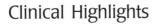

Clinical Highlights

- What aspects of a pharmacist's care plan for ambulatory patients with hypertension may require the involvement of other health care professionals?
- Which clinical conditions in ambulatory patients with hypertension require immediate attention?

Pharmaceutical care has been defined as "the responsible provision of drug therapy to achieve definite outcomes intended to improve a patient's quality of life."[1] In previous chapters, the reader has been informed of steps necessary to develop a relationship with a patient and the therapeutic options available to favorably impact the therapeutic outcome. Of equal importance for the pharmacist is an understanding of the global needs of the hypertensive patient to ensure the use of other health care providers, if appropriate. This chapter reiterates that the pharmacist is an integral member of the health care team, but it also reinforces the pharmacist's need to know when other health care providers are required to ensure implementation of treatment regimens designed to affect outcomes favorably.

The Care Plan: Involving Other Health Care Professionals

Hypertension can result in target organ damage that may require the attention of specialists in cardiology, nephrology, neurology, and ophthalmology. Many patients with hypertension might not have or may not be aware of financial and clinical resources available to ensure the successful implementation of treatment strategies. For example, many hypertensive patients have been shown to benefit from weight reduction and reduction of excess amounts of salt within the diet, and the dietitian might be integral in developing a program to accomplish this need.

A key aspect of pharmaceutical care within the framework of nutritional factors is that the pharmacy practitioner must include dietary discussions into any care plan being developed for a patient with hypertension. However, an uncommon practice, which needs to become more routine, is to have the pharmacist call upon the additional skills and training of a dietitian to follow-up with patients who either do not appreciate the importance of diet and the long-term complications of hypertension or those patients who just cannot implement the appropriate nutrition necessary to change their lifestyles.

Noncompliance with therapeutic diets remains a major obstacle to achieving improvements in cardiovascular disease morbidity and mortality.[2] A systematic team approach in utilizing all health care professionals, including the physician, pharmacist, nurse, social worker, and dietitian, increases the likelihood that a hypertensive patient will be adequately educated and monitored by those most knowledgeable in a specific area. Carefully developed personalized programs should be used to encourage lifestyle changes specific for each patient.

The seventh report of the Joint National Committee on Prevention, Detection, Evaluation, and Treatment of High Blood Pressure (JNC 7) provides guidance in the form of lifestyle modifications as a way to help prevent hypertension and to manage hypertension. Several of the lifestyle modifications center on dietary influences (**Table 9-1**).

Triage and Referral of Ambulatory Patients with Hypertension

The role the pharmacist plays in the management of hypertension is dependent on the practice environment and available resources. In a clinic setting,

Table 9-1.
Lifestyle Modifications for Hypertension Prevention and Management

1. Lose weight if overweight.
2. Limit alcohol intake to no more than 1 oz of ethanol, 24 oz of beer, 10 oz of wine, or 2 oz of 100-proof whiskey per day or 0.5 oz of ethanol per day for women and lighter weight people.
3. Increase aerobic physical activity (30–45 minutes most days of the week).
4. Reduce sodium intake to no more than 100 mmol per day (2.4 grams of sodium or 6 grams of sodium chloride).
5. Maintain adequate intake of dietary potassium (approximately 90 mmol per day).
6. Maintain adequate intake of dietary calcium and magnesium for general health.
7. Stop smoking and reduce intake of dietary saturated fat and cholesterol for overall cardiovascular health.

the pharmacist may have access to patient-specific records and laboratory information. This may provide the resources necessary for a more extensive role in the patient's care plan.

In the setting of a community pharmacy, limited resources might not allow for adequate review of patient records. The pharmacist will become more dependent on other members of the health care team to obtain the necessary information to adequately monitor a hypertensive patient's care plan. (See the section on the Health Insurance Portability and Accountability Act of 1996.)

Routine monitoring of drug therapy is a professional responsibility that all pharmacists in all settings should assume, regardless of resources. Comprehensive therapeutic monitoring, compliance, and assessing for cost-effective therapy are areas in which pharmacists must be prepared to actively participate. As mentioned in Chapter 3, the use of physical assessment skills to monitor blood pressure and the impact of drug therapy on a patient can be appropriately incorporated into daily care plans for each patient.

Discussions involving the assessment of dietary needs, ability to obtain medications, nutrition, smoking cessation, and the development of an exercise program are important aspects of a patient's care plan that can be adequately addressed by a pharmacist. However, for many hypertensive patients, a more specific focus in each of these areas

may require the pharmacist to refer to other trained professionals who may be better suited to meet the specific needs of a patient.

A pharmacist is capable of discussing the general needs of a hypertensive patient's diet. However, the dietitian is better suited to assist in detailed meal planning. Similarly, a pharmacist is able to identify opportunities for reducing costs associated with a specific therapy prescribed by a physician. However, the social worker is better suited to identify local organizations or governmental programs that might be available to provide the resources necessary to ensure availability of a patient's prescriptions.

An elderly hypertensive patient living at home may require the services of a home care provider to obtain necessary care. A social worker may be necessary in such circumstances to ensure adequate resources that would allow the hypertensive patient to remain at home rather than travel for visits with trained health care providers.

Roles of Primary Care Physicians, Specialists, and Social Workers

As hypertension progresses, target organ damage will require the skill and training of medical specialists. For many patients, initial care will be provided by a primary care physician. When a patient is unable to obtain the targeted blood pressure goal despite optimizing drug dosages and combinations, the JNC 7 guidelines recommend that consultation with hypertension specialists be considered.[2]

The pharmacist will continue to play an integral role as the provider of drug therapy in these patients. As target organ damage develops, the growing list of medications prescribed will increase the challenges for the pharmacist to monitor therapeutic effects and will expand the need for drug–drug interaction monitoring, drug–disease state interaction monitoring, and drug–medical expert communication monitoring.

The growing number of prescribers will require the need to maximize efficient communication between all health care providers and the patient. The pharmacist is the ideal person to serve as the central communication link among the growing network of health care providers.

During recent years, a growing number of states have acknowledged pharmacists as having specialized knowledge and abilities that contribute to quality patient care.[3] For many practicing pharmacists, this has resulted in the implementation of *Collaborative Practice Agreements* as a way to integrate their services with those of physicians.[4] Practice agreements, though relatively new in pharmacy, have been used for quite some time in nursing as a way to expand the role of nurses in physician practices.

A collaborative practice agreement is an agreement between a pharmacist and a prescriber that allows for an expanded level of authority by the pharmacist for certain types of activities. In the management of patients with hypertension, this might include the use of a treatment protocol where a pharmacist may be given the authority to adjust therapeutic regimens based on guidelines and protocols and preestablished treatment plans intended to optimize patient care. Collaborative practice agreements have continued to gain favor based on encouraging outcomes demonstrated by pharmacists in various types of patient care settings.

Health Insurance Portability and Accountability Act (HIPAA) of 1996

On April 14, 2003, the Department of Health and Human Services published standards that provided patients with access to their own medical records as well as providing more control over how a patient's personal health information could be used and disclosed.[5,6] A key component of HIPAA is the privacy rule, which requires health plans, pharmacies, physicians, and other health care entities to develop policies and procedures to protect the confidentiality of protected health information of patients. HIPAA affects all practicing pharmacists, both those primarily responsible for the provision of medications as well as those who are involved in clinical patient care activities. HIPAA has already had an impact on the manner in which health care information is utilized by health care providers.

As pharmacists proceed with the implementation of pharmaceutical care in hypertensive patients, a critical understanding of HIPAA is necessary to allow active participation as a member of the health care team. A lack of understanding of HIPAA by pharmacists could result in exclusionary decisions being made by others who are concerned over potential liability issues originating from HIPAA policies and procedures.

Hypertensive Crises: Urgencies and Emergencies

The ambulatory care pharmacist should be aware of the clinical scenarios of hypertensive urgency and emergency. These two clinical situations may necessitate immediate referral to other health care providers. The patient might be suffering from an urgent hypertensive situation not associated with target organ damage but which would require that the blood pressure be controlled within a 6–24-hour period. In hypertensive emergency, severely elevated blood pressure is associated with signs and symptoms of target organ damage.

In both situations, the ambulatory care pharmacist should seek input from other health care providers. In hypertensive urgency, the initial care may be provided outside of the hospital environment. As stated in the JNC 7 guidelines, it is desirable to reduce blood pressure within a few hours in order to prevent target organ damage.[7] The pharmacist would contact a physician, in most cases, the primary medical practitioner who oversees the care of the hypertensive patient. The physician is likely to request that the patient be brought to his/her office or clinic for evaluation as an outpatient.

In hypertensive emergency, the presence of acute target organ damage requires additional monitoring and immediate treatment to prevent further complications. Often this would require hospitalization of the patient to achieve this goal in a timely manner. The pharmacist would likely need to contact members of the emergency treatment services of his or her community to transport the patient to a hospital facility for quick observation and treatment.

The following situations require immediate aggressive therapeutic interventions and hospitalization: accelerated and malignant hypertension, hypertensive encephalopathy, intracranial hemorrhage, unstable angina pectoris, acute myocardial infarction, acute left ventricular dysfunction with pulmonary edema, acute aortic aneurysm, evidence of renal function deterioration, and eclampsia. Assessment must be done promptly and efficiently so that transport to the necessary environment occurs as soon as possible.

Summary

Pharmaceutical care has become the term employed to symbolize the direct impact that pharmacy practitioners have on patients within various health care settings. Today's practitioner recognizes that the provision of pharmaceutical care or more clearly stated "the responsible provision of drug therapy to achieve definite outcomes" does not routinely take place in a vacuum. It requires a collaborative effort among all members of the health care team to ensure the "improvement in a patient's quality of life."

The hypertensive patient provides a wide array of challenges to the health care team, and one of the most important is the assurance that each member of the team supports the patient care plan. There is a need for the pharmacist to be able to recognize situations that should be referred to other members of the team. As pharmacists begin to maximize communication pathways between health care providers and patients, the literature suggests that the long-term goals of improving quality of life and participating as an active member of the health care team will become commonplace throughout all health care systems.[8]

Key Points for Patients

- Pharmacists, in conjunction with primary care physicians, social workers, dietitians, and specialized physicians (cardiologists, neurologists, nephrologists, and ophthalmologists), represent key members of the hypertensive patient's health care team.

- As a member of the health care team, pharmacists are able to collaborate with other members of the team to see that all aspects of the patient's hypertension treatment are implemented appropriately.

- Collaboration and communication among members of the health care team are only possible with the active participation of the hypertensive patient. This will help to ensure that all health care providers have the necessary information to actively participate in the treatment plan.

- Each member of the health care team needs to identify those circumstances that may require other members of the team and to recognize that the ultimate goal is to maximize outcomes associated with all aspects of the patient's therapeutic regimen including diet, lifestyle modification, pharmacologic treatment, nonpharmacologic treatment, and specialized end organ treatment.

References

1. Hepler CD, Strand LM. Opportunities and responsibilities in pharmaceutical care. *Am J Hosp Pharm.* 1990; 47:533–43.

2. The seventh report of the Joint National Committee on Prevention, Detection, Evaluation, and Treatment of High Blood Pressure. The JNC 7 report. *JAMA.* 2003; 289:2560–72.

3. Collaborative practice agreements: American Society of Consultant Pharmacists; Policy statement on collaborative practice. Approved by the ASCP Board of Directors, November 11, 1997 http://www.ascp.com/public/pr/policy/collaborative.shtml. (accessed 2003 Aug 28).

4. Furo LA, Marcrom RE, Garrelts L et al. Collaborative practice agreements between pharmacists and physicians. *J Am Pharm Assoc.* 1998; 38:655–64.

5. Health and Human Services. Office for Civil Rights-HIPAA. Medical Privacy-National Standards to Protect the Privacy of Personal Health Information. www.hhs.gov/ocr/hipaa/ (accessed 2003 Aug 27).

6. Bishop SK, Winckler SC. Implementing HIPAA privacy regulations in pharmacy practice. *J Am Pharm Assoc.* 2002; 42:836–46.

7. The sixth report of the Joint National Committee on Prevention, Detection, Evaluation, and Treatment of High Blood Pressure. National Heart, Lung, and Blood Institute, National Institutes of Health, November 1997; NIH publication no. 98-4080.

8. McDonough RP, Doucette WR. Dynamics of pharmaceutical care continuing education monograph series. Collaborations between pharmacists and physicians. Steps for building more effective working relationships—monograph 19. A continuing education program sponsored by Merck and APhA. http://www.aphanet.org (accessed 2003 Aug 29).

Chapter 10:

Evaluation of Therapeutic Outcomes

Alan H. Mutnick

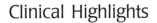

Clinical Highlights

FDA Modernization Act of 1997

Outcomes Research

Pharmacoeconomics

Decision Analysis

Literature Example

Summary

Key Points for Patients

References

Clinical Highlights

- What is the impact of the FDA Modernization Act on practicing pharmacists?
- What practical issues are important when interpreting pharmacoeconomic and outcomes research studies?
- What framework can be used for assessing the generalizability of published outcomes studies?
- What is the role of pharmacoeconomic information during the decision-making process?
- What different models and/or techniques can be used?

The growing societal concerns about costs, access, and quality of health care have required health care providers to develop methods for evaluating the respective resources needed to provide such care. The treatment of hypertension has been, and will continue to be, an area ripe for societal concerns, especially as practitioners design treatment regimens consistent with national/international guidelines, while taking into consideration costs to patients, their insurance companies, and governmental agencies.

The pharmacy profession has not been ignored in this regard. Decisions need to be made regarding the use of less costly generic drug products versus the more expensive *cutting-edge* new therapeutic agents. Is cheaper always better, or is there potential value in using an expensive drug product? Additionally, terms such as *cost-effective, cost-benefit*, and *cost-prohibitive* increasingly are used to describe the various therapies available, and such terms have also found their way into the marketing of pharmaceuticals. These terms have also been used in an effort to describe the professional value appreciated for various levels of pharmacy practice.

This final chapter provides an overview of *outcomes research* and compares and contrasts it to more traditional research involving randomized clinical trials. Additionally, an example will be provided that serves as a starting point for ways to carry out outcomes research, as well as ways to quantify the value for various types of pharmacy products and/or services. If pharmacists are not able to utilize principles of outcomes research, others will become the decision makers, and that might not be consistent with the principles set forth describing *pharmaceutical care*.

FDA Modernization Act of 1997

Section 114 of the act is referred to as Health Care Economic Information and states that:[1]

> *Health care economic information provided to a formulary committee, or other similar entity, in the course of the committee or entity carrying out its responsibilities for the selection of drugs for managed care or other similar organizations, shall not be considered to be false or misleading under this paragraph if the health care economic information directly relates to an indication approved . . . . for such drug and is based on competent and reliable scientific evidence.*

Health care economic information means any analysis that identifies, measures, or compares the economic consequences, including the costs of the represented health outcomes, or the use of a drug to the use of another drug, to another health care intervention, or to no intervention.

This portion of the Modernization Act serves as a venue for the pharmaceutical industry to provide pharmacoeconomic and outcomes research studies to decision makers. This information can be provided in the form of cost-minimization analysis (CMA), cost-effectiveness analysis (CEA), cost-benefit analysis (CBA), cost-utility analysis (CUA), cost of illness (COI), and cost-quality of life. The overall intention of Section 114 is to provide competent and reliable scientific information pertaining to a given drug's approved indication.[1]

Although Section 114 provides what many feel is beneficial information to drug formulary decision makers, it does impose certain educational requirements on them and, in particular, on pharmacy decision makers. Among the educational requirements are the following four necessary components: (1) decision makers must possess excellent knowledge on the various pharmacoeconomic techniques utilized by the pharmaceutical industry; (2) decision makers must have the ability to evaluate studies to identify the most cost-effective strategy or therapy utilized; (3) decision makers must be able to educate prescribers on the various studies and be able to point out the biases and limitations; and (4) decision makers need to be able to perform such various types of pharmacoeconomic analyses using regional/local data to allow finalization of decisions. In the remaining portions of this chapter, the reader will be introduced to the different aspects of outcomes research and pharmacoeconomics to become better able to analyze, evaluate, and implement such studies.

Outcomes Research

Outcomes research (OR) is broadly defined as research that identifies, measures, and evaluates the end results of health care services in terms of clinical, economic, and humanistic consequences.[2] More specifically, OR is the study of health care interventions (treatment modalities such as drug therapies, surgery, or palliative therapy), care delivery processes, and health care quality that are evaluated to measure the extent to which optimal and desirable outcomes can be reached.

Normally, the purpose of OR is to assess the *value* of a program or therapy in question, and the concept of value forms the foundation for the model. In order to assess the value of a treatment, or to compare the value of opposing treatment alternatives, all three types of outcomes should be considered. It is also important to recognize that many

of the actual outcomes themselves overlap. For example, many clinical outcomes are measurable on humanistic scales (such as pain, a clinical outcome, measured on a visual analog pain scale).

The economic, clinical, and humanistic outcomes (ECHO) model was introduced as a means to evaluate the value of pharmaceutical products or services by integrating the more traditional clinical-based outcomes with contemporary measures of economics and quality.[2] By employing the ECHO model, decision makers are better able to evaluate systematically by considering the benefits/risks among economic, clinical, and humanistic outcomes to make more informed comprehensive decisions from a more multidimensional perspective (**Table 10-1**). OR methodologies include retrospective chart review, prospective clinical trials, observational studies, and computer-modeling studies.

Much confusion exists in comparing and contrasting OR from the more traditional randomized clinical trials. The purpose of OR is to supplement rather than replace controlled clinical trials. Although similar to randomized clinical trials, OR is research with different intentions than those found in randomized clinical trials (**Table 10-2**).

Table 10-1.
Types of Outcomes Associated with the ECHO Model

Economic
- Acquisition costs associated with the provision of care
- Labor costs associated with the provision of care
- Costs associated with the treatment of adverse drug reactions—acute and long term
- Costs associated with treatment failure—acute and long term
- Costs associated with readmission to hospital
- Costs associated with emergency room and clinic visits

Clinical
- Length of hospital stay
- Hospital admission and/or readmission rates
- Emergency room and/or clinic visits
- Rates of development of adverse drug reactions
- Death

Humanistic
- Functional status measured by a validated instrument
- Quality of life measured by a validated instrument
- Patient satisfaction with care provided

Table 10-2.

Comparison between OR and Randomized Clinical Trials (RCT)

Characteristics associated with OR	Characteristics of RCT
Cost effectiveness	Evaluation of clinical efficacy to determine if a given therapy works
Generalized to a broader patient population likely to receive the drug product under normal daily living conditions	Restrictions placed on entry criteria to create very specific and distinct patient population
Large sample size	Relatively small sample size
Observational study	Strict experimental design

Pharmacoeconomics

Pharmacoeconomics (PE) is the science of measuring the costs and outcomes associated with the use of pharmaceuticals in health care delivery. PE is a tool, not the solution, for decision makers. It is used with OR and utilizes different types of mathematical models and techniques to compare the costs and effectiveness of drugs; to select clinical services, disease state management pathways, and medical/surgical devices; and to allow decision makers to determine value. PE research identifies, measures, and compares the costs (resources consumed) and consequences (clinical, economic, and humanistic) of pharmaceutical products and services.

The science of PE has seen the development of several methodologies frequently utilized to carry out the analysis, i.e., COI, CBA, CMA, CEA, CUA, and willingness to pay. Each methodology provides specific types of information and is dependent on designated rules and guidelines to provide the greatest information to decision makers (**Table 10-3**).

For some who become involved for the first time in OR or PE studies, there is a striking difference between the types of research methods utilized as compared to those frequently used during the more traditional randomized clinical trials. However, an important distinction between the purposes of these two types of studies should clarify such differences (Table 10-2). Randomized clinical trials provide the fundamental basis for drug product evaluations in a very structured, carefully defined fashion. The evaluations are based on very specific inclusion and exclusion criteria and rely on a sample of preselected patient populations presenting with a minimal number of differentiating characteristics in order to assure a homogeneous population directly affected by a specific study intervention. Most experts would agree that this type of study is necessary to evaluate the clinical value or *efficacy* of a particular product anticipated to be marketed for a specific disease process or ailment.

OR evaluates a drug product or clinical service for its impact in the real-world setting, with all the constraints, distractions, and experiences of real daily living among a larger population of typical people who might receive such a treatment. Randomized clinical trials might reveal data that an antihypertensive medication is a very efficacious drug when administered three times daily, perhaps 1 hour before meals. OR might demonstrate that the general population trying to take the medication three times daily, 1 hour before meals is unable to be compliant with the regimen, and consequently the *effectiveness* of the drug might be less than anticipated, in the real-world environment. Properly designed OR or PE studies are able to provide very useful information about drug products and clinical services by affording more generalizability to entire populations as compared to the limited applicability of most randomized clinical trials.

Decision Analysis

Decision analysis is one tool that has been used in carrying out OR and represents a systematic approach to making decisions under conditions of uncertainty. It utilizes various techniques as aids in analyzing situations and requires the decision maker to outline the decision, to identify and evaluate the consequences of outcomes, and to then assign values to each possible outcome.[3] The major components involved in carrying out decision analysis include the following six steps:

1. Determine the decision alternatives.
2. Structure the decision process.
3. Assess the probability for each respective outcome.

Table 10-3.
Types of Pharmacoeconomic Methodologies

Methodology	Description	Purpose
Cost of Illness (COI)	Evaluation and assessment of the resources necessary to treat an illness.	Used to obtain baseline cost information prior to the assessment of a potentially new intervention.
Cost–Benefit Analysis (CBA)	Evaluation used to determine the priorities for dedicating resource allocation.	Used to compare programs as well as specific interventions by evaluating costs (dollars) and their associated benefits.
Cost-Minimization Analysis (CMA)	Evaluation involves the different costs associated with each therapeutic intervention recognizing that outcomes are equivalent.	Many formulary decisions made by Pharmacy & Therapeutics Committees are based on this methodology where the outcome is not in question, but rather the costs associated with achieving the respective outcomes.
Cost-Effectiveness Analysis (CEA)	Evaluation used to measure a single outcome in natural units relevant to changes in mortality or morbidity.	Used to assist in identifying a preferred choice among possible alternatives with similar consequences (e.g., same therapeutic category) in terms of health improvement created (e.g., life year gained, clinical cures).
Cost-Utility Analysis (CUA)	The measurement of the consequences of an intervention in terms of quality	Employed to provide an assessment of the costs expended as a function of the health state obtained; the results are expressed as the costs per quality-adjusted life year (QALY).
Willingness to Pay (WTP)	Evaluation that takes into account the psychological aspects of a given illness as well as the physical deterioration; provides a means to assign dollar values to health outcomes.	Used to assess the perceived value or benefit of a drug product or select service.

4. Determine the value of each outcome.

5. Select the decision alternative with desired expected value.

6. Conduct a sensitivity analysis.

Numerous examples are available in the peer-reviewed literature and are provided in the Decision Analysis section of **Appendix 10-1**.

Literature Example

The Heart Outcomes Prevention Evaluation Study (HOPE) was initiated in 1993.[4] HOPE recruited 9297 male and female patients who were randomized to receive either ramipril 10 mg daily or placebo to evaluate the prevention of the primary endpoint, a composite of cardiovascular death, myocardial infarction, and stroke. HOPE was not a blood pressure study, and the inclusion criteria did not include hypertension and specifically excluded heart failure, both usual indications for ACE inhibitors. The trial did not consider economic endpoints relevant to U.S. decision makers.

More than half of the patients entered into the study had no history of hypertension, and those who did were required to be controlled on medications prior to study entry. The mean blood pressure of all patients at study entry was 139/79. The majority of patients in the HOPE study were receiving concomitant therapy for cardiovascular conditions at time of entry and throughout the study. Therefore, the benefit of ramipril was in addition to other *usual care* therapies, many of which have already been shown to improve outcomes. Ramipril resulted in a 22% reduction over placebo in cardiovascular mortality, myocardial infarction, and stroke.

Recently, an attempt was made to provide a tool to assist U.S. decision makers by analyzing the 2- and 4-year economic implications of the HOPE study. The study was referred to as the cost of prevention economic (COPE) model and is an example of integrating clinical outcomes data with the financial consequences associated with the decision-making process[5] (**Figure 10-1**).

The COPE model utilized data from the literature[6–8] to quantify the costs associated with the treatment of stroke, myocardial infarction, percutaneous transluminal coronary angioplasty, coronary artery bypass grafting, and congestive heart failure along with the clinical outcomes presented in the HOPE trial. The model demonstrated that

Figure 10-1.
An Example of a Decision Model Utilizing the HOPE Study

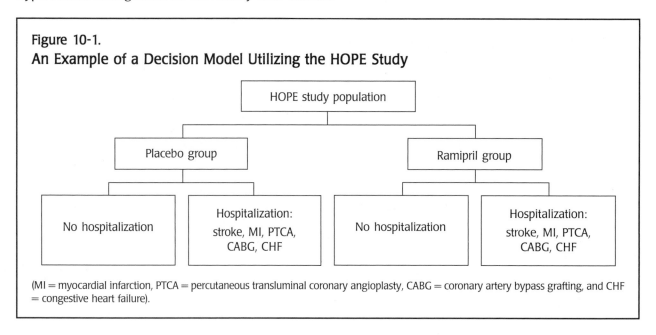

(MI = myocardial infarction, PTCA = percutaneous transluminal coronary angioplasty, CABG = coronary artery bypass grafting, and CHF = congestive heart failure).

over a 4-year period the use of ramipril resulted in the avoidance of 294 clinical events (stroke, myocardial infarction, congestive heart failure, etc.) based on the findings from the HOPE trial, and it found a net savings of $767,665 for the more than 9,000 patients ($1.76 per member per month savings over the 4-year period) included in the HOPE trial, based on the clinical event costs identified from the literature.[6–8] Net savings refer to the savings appreciated after spending on all health care resources including patient hospitalizations, clinic visits, physician visits, medications, etc.

Summary

The treatment of hypertension relies on more than the use of inexpensive medications to treat the patient. Outcomes research and pharmacoeconomics remove the *silo* mentality from the decision-making process to allow decision makers to look beyond drug price in order to render an accurate decision. The implementation of the FDA Modernization Act of 1997 has provided the pharmaceutical industry with a venue to communicate with decision makers on the clinical, economic, and humanistic outcomes associated with drug therapy.

If pharmacists are going to participate in making informed decisions regarding drug therapy selection in hypertensive patients, interest and, in many cases, the ability to evaluate, analyze, and implement outcomes-type research will be necessary. If pharmacists are not able to carry out these functions adequately, future decisions will be left in the hands of those most able to interpret the information provided by industry representatives, and the opportunity to contribute in this vital area will be lost.

Key Points for Patients

- There are numerous medications available for the treatment of hypertension, but, by utilizing the literature, specific drugs can be identified that are most likely to help a patient achieve his or her blood pressure goal with the least number of adverse effects at the lowest cost.
- Sometimes, medications that have low costs turn out to be the best medications for hypertension treatment as they also have low incidence of side effects and are able to achieve the blood pressure goal. However, in some instances, the least expensive medication might not achieve the blood pressure goal or it might have a higher incidence of side effects than a medication that costs more.
- The goal of hypertension management is to design the most effective therapeutic regimen for achieving the target blood pressure goal while causing the fewest side effects at the lowest overall costs.
- Costs of hypertension treatment include more than the cost of the medications and include the costs of medication side effects and hospitalizations for medical problems caused by hypertension, etc.

References

1. FDA Modernization Act of 1997. http://www.fda.gov/cdrh/modact/modern.html (accessed 2003 February 15).

2. Kozma CM, Reeder CE, Schulz RM. Economic, clinical, and humanistic outcomes: a planning model for pharmacoeconomic research. *Clin Ther.* 1993; 15(6): 1121–32.

3. Barr JT, Schumacher GE. Decision analysis and pharmacoeconomic evaluations. In: Principles of Pharmacoeconomics. Bootman JL, Townsend RJ, McGhan WF, eds. Cincinnati: Harvey Whitney Books; 1991.

4. Yusuf S, Sleight P, Pogue J et al. Effects of an angiotensin-converting-enzyme inhibitor, ramipril, on cardiovascular events in high-risk patients. The Heart Outcomes Prevention Evaluation Study Investigators (HOPE). *N Engl J Med.* 2000; 342:145–53.

5. Carroll C. Cost of prevention evaluation (COPE) training manual. November 2000.

6. Holloway RG, Witter DM, Lawton KB et al. Inpatient costs of specific cerebrovascular events at five academic medical centers. *Neurology.* 1996; 46:854–60.

7. Krumholz HM, Chen J, Murillo JE et al. Clinical correlates of in-hospital costs for acute myocardial infarction in patients 65 years of age and older. *Am Heart J.* 1998; 135:523–31.

8. Bennett SJ, Saywell RM, Zollinger TW et al. Cost of hospitalizations for heart failure: sodium retention versus other decompensating factors. *Heart Lung.* 1999; 28:102–9.

Appendix 10-1.
Suggested Readings

General Texts and References on Outcomes Research and Pharmacoeconomics

1. Bootman JL, Townsend RJ, McGhan WF, eds. Principles of pharmacoeconomics. Cincinnati: Harvey Whitney Books; 1996.

2. Bungay KM, Osterhaus JT, Paladino JA et al. Pharmacoeconomics and outcomes: applications for patient care. Kansas City, MO: American College of Clinical Pharmacy; 1996. NOTE: This series of binders comprises a self-study program marketed by ACCP. It is an excellent starting point for more detailed, self-study of this topic.

3. Drummond MF, Stoddard GL, Torrance GW. Methods for the economic evaluation of health care programmes. Oxford, England: Oxford University Press; 1987.

4. Gold MR, Siegel JE, Russell LB et al., eds. Cost-effectiveness in health and medicine. New York: Oxford University Press; 1996.

Outcomes as a Pharmacy Leadership Skill

1. Gouveia WA. Applying patient outcomes and pharmacoeconomics in patient care. Am J Health Syst Pharm. 1995; 52 (14 Suppl 3):S11–5.

2. Johannesson M. Economic evaluation of drugs and its potential uses in policy making. Pharmacoeconomics. 1995; 8:190–8.

3. McCombs JS, Nichol MB, Johnson KA et al. Is pharmacy's vision of the future too narrow? Am J Health Syst Pharm. 1995; 52:1208–14.

4. McGhan WF, Briesacher BA. Implementing pharmacoeconomic outcomes management. Pharmacoeconomics. 1994; 6:412–6.

5. Mutnick AH, Sterba KJ, Szymusiak-Mutnick BA. The integration of quality assessment and a patient-specific intervention/outcomes program. Pharm Pract Manage Q. 1998; 17(4):25–36.

6. Sanchez LA. Expanding the role of the pharmacist in pharmacoeconomics: how and why? Pharmacoeconomics. 1994; 5:367–75.

Outcomes in Drug Use Evaluation and Formulary Management

1. Angaran DM. Selecting, developing, and evaluating indicators. Am J Hosp Pharm. 1991; 48:1931–7.

2. Becker AJ, Mutnick AH, Ross MB et al. Combining a clinical trial with decision analysis to evaluate antiemetic agents. Formulary. 1996; 31:670–86.

3. Hatoum HT, Freeman RA. The use of pharmacoeconomic data in formulary selection. Top Hosp Pharm Manage. 1994; 13:47–53.

4. Schrogie JJ, Nash DB. Relationship between practice guidelines, formulary management, and pharmacoeconomic studies. Top Hosp Pharm Manage. 1994; 13:38–46.

5. Szymusiak-Mutnick BA, Mutnick AH. An application of decision analysis in antibiotic formulary choices. J Pharm Technol. 1994; 10:23–6.

Decision Analysis

1. Barr JT, Schumacher GE. Applying decision analysis to pharmacy management and practice decisions. Top Hosp Pharm Manage. 1994; 14:60–71.

2. Detsky AS, Naglie G, Krahn MD et al. Primer on medical decision analysis: part 2—building a tree. Med Decis Making. 1997; 17:126–35.

3. Detsky AS, Naglie G, Krahn MD et al. Primer on medical decision analysis: part 1—getting started. Med Decis Making. 1997; 17:123–5.

4. Krahn MD, Naglie G, Naimark D et al. Primer on medical decision analysis: part 4—analyzing the model and interpreting the results. Med Decis Making. 1997; 17:142–51.

5. Naglie G, Krahn MD, Naimark D et al. Primer on medical decision analysis: part 3—estimating probabilities and utilities. Med Decis Making. 1997; 17:136–41.

6. Naimark D, Krahn MD, Naglie G et al. Primer on medical decision analysis: part 5—working with Markov processes. Med Decis Making. 1997; 17:152–9.

Evaluating, Interpreting, and Communicating Results of Outcomes Research Studies

1. Drummond MF, Richardson WS, O'Brien BJ et al. Users' guideline to the medical literature. XIII. How to use an article on economic analysis of clinical practice. A. Are the results of the study valid? JAMA. 1997; 277:1552–7.

2. Hay JW. Comment re: evaluation of pharmacoeconomic studies: utilization of a checklist [letter]. Ann Pharmacother. 1994; 28:539.

3. Hillman AL, Eisenberg JM, Pauly MV et al. Avoiding bias in the conduct and reporting of cost-effectiveness research sponsored by pharmaceutical companies. N Engl J Med. 1991; 324:1362–5.

4. Jacobs P, Bachynsky J, Baladi JF. A comparative review of pharmacoeconomics guidelines. Pharmacoeconomics. 1995; 8:182–9.

5. Johnson N. Translating and implementing outcomes research into clinical practice. Formulary. 1999; 34:251–6.

6. Jolicoeur LM, Jones-Grizzle AJ, Boyer JG. Guidelines for performing a pharmacoeconomic analysis. Am J Hosp Pharm. 1992; 49:741–7.

7. O'Brien BJ, Heyland D, Richardson WS et al. Users' guideline to the medical literature. XIII. How to use an article on economic analysis of clinical practice. B. What are the results and will they help me in caring for my patients? JAMA. 1997; 277:1802–6.

8. Redelmeier DA, Detsky AS, Krahn MD et al. Guidelines for verbal presentations of medical decision analyses. Med Decis Making. 1997; 17:228–30.

9. Sacristan JA, Soto J, Galende I. Evaluation of pharmacoeconomic studies: utilization of a checklist. Ann Pharmacother. 1993; 27:1126–33.

10. Sanchez LA. Applied pharmacoeconomics: Evaluation and use of pharmacoeconomic data from the literature. Am J Health Syst Pharm. 1999; 56:1630–40.

11. Schulman KA, Rubenstein LE, Glick HA et al. Relationships between sponsors and investigators in pharmacoeconomic and clinical research. *Pharmacoeconomics.* 1995; 7:206–20.

12. Siegel JE, Torrance GW, Russell LB et al. Guidelines for pharmacoeconomic studies: recommendations from the Panel on Cost Effectiveness in Health and Medicine. *Pharmacoeconomics.* 1997; 11:159–68.

13. Trakas K, Addis A, Kruk D et al. Quality assessment of pharmacoeconomic abstracts of original research articles in selected journals. *Ann Pharmacother.* 1997; 31:423–8.

General Outcomes, Health Services Research Methods

1. D'Agostino RB, Kwan H. Measuring effectiveness: What to expect without a randomized control group. *Med Care.* 1995; 44(Suppl):AS95–AS105.

2. Gandhi SK, Salmon JW, Kong SX et al. Administrative databases and outcomes assessment: an overview of issues and potential utility. *J Managed Care Pharm.* 1999; 5:215–22.

3. Hillman AL, Kim MS. Economic decision making in healthcare: a standard approach to discounting health outcomes. *Pharmacoeconomics.* 1995; 7:198–205.

4. Hurley SF. Indices of therapeutic outcome in pharmacoeconomic evaluation of drug therapy. *Pharmacoeconomics.* 1992; 1:155–60.

5. Johnson NE, Tsai WW. Pharmacoeconomic outcomes studies vs randomized clinical trials. *P&T.* 1994; 19:84–9.

6. Kozma CM, Reeder CE, Schulz RM. Economic, clinical, and humanistic outcomes: a planning model for pharmacoeconomic research. *Clin Ther.* 1993; 15:1121–32.

7. Mason J. The generalizability of pharmacoeconomic studies. *Pharmacoeconomics.* 1997; 11:503–14.

8. McCoy S, Blayney-Chandramouli J, Mutnick A. Using multiple pharmacoeconomic models to conduct a cost-effectiveness analysis of histamine H_2 receptor antagonists. *Am J Health Syst Pharm.* 1998; 55(Suppl): S8–S12.

9. McPherson K. The best and the enemy of the good: randomised controlled trials, uncertainty, and assessing the role of patient choice in medical decision making. *J Epidemiol Community Health.* 1994; 48:6–15.

10. Miller DW. The impact of methodological and drug development issues on the use of economic data generated by clinical trials. *Pharm Pract Manage Q.* 1997; 17:75–86.

11. Rubenstein EB, Elting LS. Pharmacoeconomic analyses: Whose perspective counts and costs the most? *Am J Hosp Pharm.* 1994; 51:564–9.

12. Stewart LA, Parmar MK. Bias in the analysis and reporting of randomized controlled trials. *Int J Technol Assess Health Care.* 1996; 12:264–75.

13. Smith TA, Dillon DM, Kotula RJ et al. Evaluation of antimicrobial surgical prophylaxis with multiattribute utility theory. *Am J Health Syst Pharm.* 2001; 58:251–5.

Quality-of-Life Assessment

1. Erickson P, Taeuber RC, Scott J. Operational aspects of quality-of-life assessment. Choosing the right instrument. *Pharmacoeconomics.* 1995; 7:39–48.

2. Leplege A, Hunt S. The problem of quality of life in medicine. *JAMA.* 1997; 278:47–50.

3. Testa MA, Simonson DC. Assessment of quality-of-life outcomes. *N Engl J Med.* 1996; 334:835–40.

Continuing Education

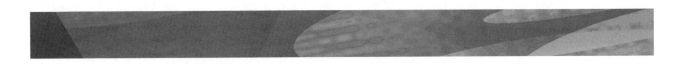

Dear Purchaser:

To complete the CE program for this product, go to the ASHP CE Testing Center at **http://www.ashp. org/ce/**. Log in using your Customer ID Number from the purchase invoice or your ASHP Member ID Number. Once you have successfully logged in, follow the instructions provided for completing and submitting your test. Thank you.

CE process

The continuing-education (CE) test for this book can only be taken online through ASHP's CE Testing Center. If you score 70% or better on the test, you will be able to immediately print your own CE statement for your records. You will have two opportunities to pass the CE test, and you may stop and return to the test at any time before submitting your final answers. ASHP will keep a record of the credits you have earned from this and other CE activities, and you will be able to view your own transcript through the online CE service.

Title: Hypertension Management for the Primary Care Clinician

ACPE#: 204-000-04-043-H04

CE credit: 7.0 hours

Expiration date: April 30, 2007

Instructions

ASHP members may go directly to www.ashp.org/ce/, select "Register for Test," and then select the article for which CE credit is desired. CE is $20.95 per test for members.

Nonmembers must go to the ASHP Shopping Cart (www.ashp.org/products-services), select "Browse Online Catalog," select "Products" in the navigation bar, and select "Continuing Education." The fee for non-ASHP members is $30.95 per test.

Questions? Call ASHP Customer Service at 301-657-4383.

The American Society of Health-System Pharmacists has been accredited by the American Council for Pharmacy Education as a provider of continuing pharmaceutical education.

Chapter 1

1. What percentage of hypertension patients are unaware that they have the disease?

   a. 25%

   b. 33%

   c. 50%

   d. 75%

2. Hypertension is currently controlled in what percentage of patients?

   a. 25%

   b. 32%

   c. 50%

   d. 60%

3. A group associated with a higher than average incidence of hypertension includes

   a. Mexican-Americans

   b. Caucasians

   c. Residents of the southeastern United States

   d. Males under the age of 50

4. What racial or ethnic group seems to be most affected by hypertension in the United States?

   a. Mexican-Americans

   b. Caucasians

   c. Asians

   d. African-Americans

5. The incidence of hypertension after 55 years of age is higher in women than men.

   a. True

   b. False

6. Which factor(s) further increases the risk of cardiovascular events in the setting of hypertension?

   a. Tobacco use

   b. Diabetes

   c. Age less than 50

   d. Both a and b

Chapter 2

1. Essential hypertension can be best defined as hypertension caused by
   a. Multiple factors
   b. No single cause can be identified
   c. Genetic factors
   d. Central obesity

2. What percentage of people with high blood pressure have essential, as opposed to secondary, hypertension?
   a. 50%
   b. 60%
   c. 75%
   d. 90%

3. Intake of which of the following correlates inversely with the prevalence of hypertension?
   a. Potassium
   b. Calcium
   c. Magnesium
   d. Both a and b

4. Which of the following is listed as a contributing factor to hypertension?
   a. Pollution
   b. Food additives
   c. Psychological stress
   d. Attitude

5. Screening for secondary hypertension should be conducted when which of the following clues are present?
   a. Severe hypertension
   b. Onset of high blood pressure before age 30 and after age 60
   c. Inconsistent response to therapy
   d. Variable pressures with bradycardia

6. Diastolic blood pressure is a better predictor of cardiovascular risk than systolic blood pressure.
   a. True
   b. False

7. Pulse pressure is a poor predictor of cardiovascular risk.
   a. True
   b. False

8. Consequences of uncontrolled hypertension primarily affect which of the following sites?
   a. Cardiovascular system
   b. Liver
   c. Brain
   d. Both a and c

9. Which of the following occurs first in retinopathy induced by hypertension and arteriosclerosis?
   a. Arteriovenous nicking
   b. Narrowing of the arteriolar lumen
   c. Rupturing of small vessels
   d. Swelling of the optic disk

10. End-stage renal disease associated with hypertension is most common in what ethnic/racial group?
    a. Caucasian
    b. Hispanic
    c. African-American
    d. Asian

Chapter 3

1. The medical history of a hypertension patient should include all of the following *except*
   a. Complete medication history
   b. Presence of target organ damage
   c. Illicit drug use
   d. Catecholamine levels to rule out pheochromocytoma

2. Ideally, what instrument(s) should be used to measure blood pressure?
   a. Mercury sphygmomanometer and stethoscope
   b. Calibrated aneroid manometer
   c. Validated electronic device
   d. Sphygmomanometer and right hand to feel pulse

3. Loss of flexibility of the arterial walls is the usual cause of which of the following conditions?
   a. Arrhythmia
   b. Pseudohypertension
   c. Pulsus paradoxus
   d. Orthostatic hypotension

4. Finger monitors are recommended for home use.
   a. True
   b. False

5. Tachycardia indicates how many heart beats per minute?
   a. Between 60 and 100
   b. Less than 60
   c. More than 100
   d. Between 70 and 90

6. Which of the following is not true of retinal artery findings in hypertension patients?
   a. The arterial wall is transparent.
   b. The arteries may show areas of focal or generalized narrowing.
   c. Exudates may be apparent.
   d. Hemorrhages may occur.

7. A neurological examination of a hypertension patient should include all of the following *except*
   a. Mental status
   b. Coordination and gait
   c. Intelligence testing
   d. Sensory assessment

8. Listening for "bruits" upon auscultation is helpful in monitoring for
   a. Signs of arterial narrowing
   b. Risk of stroke
   c. Labored breathing
   d. Both a and b

9. Potassium plays an active role in which of the following?
   a. Muscle relaxation
   b. Determining bone density
   c. Cardiovascular response to stress
   d. Aldosterone secretion

10. Increases in serum creatinine do *not* typically occur until more than what percentage of renal function is lost?
    a. 30%
    b. 50%
    c. 75%
    d. 90%

11. Excessive numbers of red blood cells could indicate the presence of
    a. Renal necrosis
    b. Renal tumor
    c. Kidney stones
    d. Both b and c

12. A fasting plasma glucose $\geq$126 mg/dl is the only way to reliably diagnose diabetes mellitus.
    a. True
    b. False

13. Which of the following may indicate a secondary cause of hypertension?

   a. Gradual onset of hypertension

   b. Hypertension >160/90

   c. Hypertension >180/110

   d. Hypertension that is difficult to control despite maximal medical therapy

   e. Both c and d

Chapter 4

1. Cigarette smoking increases the risk for fatal CHD by what percentage?

   a. 25%

   b. 50%

   c. 70%

   d. 80%

2. Higher rates of CHD in the elderly are likely due to

   a. Atherosclerotic changes with age

   b. Higher rates of diabetes that occur with aging

   c. Higher rates of systolic hypertension in the elderly

   d. Poor response to ACE inhibitors in patients over age 65

3. Men with a waist circumference of how many inches have an increased risk of obesity-associated complications?

   a. >30

   b. >35

   c. >40

   d. >45

4. Which of the following has been shown to lower homocysteine levels?

   a. Niacin

   b. Dietary consumption and supplementation with B vitamins

   c. Ticlopidine

   d. Gemfibrozil

5. JNC 7 and the American Diabetes Association differ in their target blood pressure recommendations for diabetics.

   a. True

   b. False

6. When aspirin is used for primary prevention of myocardial infarction in patients with hypertension, which of the following is true?

   a. The blood pressure lowering medications may be less effective.

   b. The patient should receive an H2-receptor blocker to protect against ulcers.

   c. The risk of hemorrhagic stroke may be increased if hypertension is uncontrolled.

7. What is the target HbA1c when treating diabetes?

   a. <6%

   b. <7%

   c. <8%

   d. None of the above

MS is a 51-year-old WM with a new diagnosis of hypertension, GERD, and a strong family history of CAD (father died at age 49 of MI). He works as an executive and reports high stress levels at work. He does not smoke or exercise regularly, but he does drink alcohol on a regular basis (1 drink every evening). His current medications include ASA 81 mg QD and omeprazole 20 mg QD. Blood pressure today is 150/90, heart rate 80 bpm. He weighs 100 kg at a height of 179 cm.

A lipid panel done last week revealed the following:

- Total cholesterol 234 mg/dl
- Triglycerides 195 mg/dl
- HDL 39 mg/dl
- LDL (calculated) 156 mg/dl
- Fasting blood glucose 100 mg/dl

8. Which of the following is not considered a CHD risk factor in this patient?

   a. Hypertension

   b. Family history

   c. Alcohol use

   d. Dyslipidemia

9. What is this patient's blood pressure goal?

   a. <120/80

   b. <125/85

   c. <130/85

   d. <140/90

10. What is his LDL goal?
    a. <100 mg/dl
    b. <130 mg/dl
    c. <160 mg/dl
    d. <190 mg/dl

11. What weight category does this patient belong to?
    a. Ideal
    b. Overweight
    c. Obese
    d. Severely obese

Chapter 5

1. What percentage of antihypertensive treatment regimens are changed and/or discontinued within the first 6 months?

    a. 5–10%

    b. 10–20%

    c. 25–50%

    d. 50–70%

2. The core of the treatment algorithm, developed as part of the JNC 7 guidelines, is

    a. Use of thiazide-type diuretics for the treatment of uncomplicated hypertension

    b. Initial two drug therapy if SBP >140 mmHg

    c. Use of beta blockers in diabetics as initial therapy

    d. Both a and b

3. ACEIs are recommended in the JNC 7 guidelines as first-line antihypertensive agents for uncomplicated hypertension.

    a. True

    b. False

4. Which of the following is true of AT_1 receptor antagonists?

    a. They produce a cough.

    b. They do not produce a cough.

    c. Difficulty swallowing may be a side effect.

    d. Potassium levels must be closely monitored.

5. The pharmacologic effects of doxazosin, prazosin, and terazosin are believed to be due to

    a. Blockade of the central postsynaptic α_1-receptor

    b. Direct peripheral vasodilation

    c. Blockade of the peripheral post-synaptic α_1-receptor

    d. Blockade of the peripheral post-synaptic α_2 receptor

6. Which of the following is true of relatively cardioselective β-blocking agents?

    a. Cardioselectivity is lost at higher doses, and blockade of other β-receptors will occur.

    b. They have their predominant effect on the β_1-receptor within cardiac tissue, resulting in reduced heart rate and little effect on other β-receptors.

    c. At higher doses, these agents will also block α-receptors.

    d. Both a and b

7. Which of the following is true of short-acting nifedipine?

    a. It is recommended as a first line hypertensive agent.

    b. It is recommended for use with patients with documented myocardial ischemia.

    c. It must be used with extreme caution due to association with ischemic events.

    d. It is well tolerated and has few adverse effects.

8. Which of the following is true of calcium channel blockers?

    a. They are considered alternative drugs for the initial treatment of hypertension in select patient populations unable to take diuretics or in patients with compelling indications.

    b. They all have similar adverse effect profiles.

    c. Gingival hyperplasia is a known side effect.

    d. Both a and c

9. Which class of diuretics is preferred in the treatment of hypertension?

    a. Thiazide and related diuretics

    b. Loop diuretics

    c. Potassium-sparing diuretics

10. Adverse reactions most notably associated with the three classes of diuretics involve

    a. Hypercalcemia

    b. Ototoxicity

    c. Dehydration

    d. Abnormalities in fluid and electrolyte balance

11. Which of the following is true of loop diuretics?

    a. They are considered the least potent of the diuretics.

    b. They decrease the rate of delivery of fluid and electrolytes within the renal tubule.

    c. They prevent a contraction in the plasma volume.

    d. They reduce the reabsorption of sodium by blocking the sodium-potassium-chloride transporter.

12. Use of reserpine in treating mild to moderate hypertension has significantly decreased due to

    a. Lack of efficacy in reducing hypertension

    b. High cost

    c. Potential suicidal effects

    d. Weight gain as a side effect

Chapter 6

1. Gynoid obesity is associated with a greater incidence of hypertension when compared with android obesity.

   a. True

   b. False

2. What BMI is generally considered a reasonable upper limit of healthy weight?

   a. 20

   b. 25

   c. 28

   d. 30

3. Regular aerobic exercise is essential in the maintenance of weight loss but does not otherwise contribute to controlling blood pressure.

   a. True

   b. False

4. Which group does *not* appear to have increased sensitivity to changes in dietary sodium intake?

   a. Asian heritage

   b. African-American heritage

   c. Elderly

   d. Obese

5. JNC 7 recommendations include reducing sodium intake to less than how many grams of sodium per day?

   a. 1.5

   b. 2.0

   c. 2.4

   d. 2.8

6. Hypertensive patients who are drinkers should limit their alcohol intake to how many ounces per day?

   a. .5

   b. 1

   c. 1.5

   d. 2

7. Smoking cessation aids do not elevate blood pressure because

   a. They do not contain nicotine.

   b. They contain lower doses of nicotine than cigarettes.

   c. They contain compounds that counteract the effects of nicotine.

   d. Smoking cessation aids do elevate blood pressure.

8. Caffeine should not be ingested for how many minutes prior to blood pressure evaluation?

   a. 15

   b. 30

   c. 45

   d. 60

9. JNC 7 guidelines recommend treatment with which of the following for initial choice therapy for uncomplicated hypertension, unless contraindicated?

   a. Diuretic

   b. Beta blocker

   c. ACE inhibitor

   d. Both a and b

10. Which of the following is no longer recommended for the initial treatment of hypertension?

    a. Enalapril

    b. Metoprolol

    c. Diltiazem

    d. Doxazosin

11. Different treatment approaches are necessary for hypertensive men and women.

    a. True

    b. False

12. Beta blockers are contraindicated in patients with which of the following conditions?

    a. Depression

    b. Reactive airway disease

    c. GERD

    d. Neurological disorders

SJ is a 66-year-old BF with a history of hypertension, angina, and hyperlipidemia. She is following lifestyle medication recommendations and has been able to lose weight (current BMI 24 kg/m²). Current medications include HCTZ 25 mg QD, atenolol 50 mg QD, simvastatin 40 mg QHS, Isosorbide dinitrate 20 mg TID, ASA 325 mg QD, and s/l NTG 0.4 mg prn chest pain. Her blood pressure at home continues to be above the target level and ranges from 150–160/90–95 mm Hg. Blood pressure today is 155/90 mm Hg, heart rate is 60 bpm. An electrolyte panel done last month revealed normal renal function (SrCr 1.0 mg/dl).

13. What additional antihypertensive therapy would you recommend for this patient?

   b. Captopril 25 mg TID
   c. Lisinopril 10 mg QD
   d. Diltiazem SR 180 mg QD
   e. Change HCTZ to HCTZ/Triamterene combination therapy

MM is a 80-year-old WF with a history of osteoarthritis, atrial fibrillation, hypertension, and depression. Her medications include warfarin (dose adjusted based on INR), acetaminophen 750 mg TID, capsaicin cream applied to knees BID, digoxin 0.125 mg QD, diltiazem SR 240 mg QD, and paroxetine 10 mg QD. She presents today with a blood pressure reading of 160/70 mm Hg. Her heart rate is 58 bpm. These measurements are consistent with the last few appointments she has had with her physician. She is not willing to check readings at home because she feels it is too complicated.

14. What would be an appropriate next medication to add in this clinical situation?

   a. Atenolol 25 mg QD
   b. HCTZ 12.5 mg QD
   c. HCTZ 25 mg QD
   d. Enalapril 10 mg QD

Chapter 7

1. Education of hypertension patients does *not* need to include recognizing the signs of target organ damage since this will be monitored by health care professionals.

   a. True

   b. False

2. What should the exercise recommendations be for hypertension patients?

   a. Low-level exercise for 30 minutes three times a week.

   b. Low-level exercise for an hour at least five days a week.

   c. Moderate-level exercise for 30 minutes two or three times a week.

   d. Moderate-level exercise for 30 minutes at least several times a week.

3. Herbal therapies may adversely affect blood pressure.

   a. True

   b. False

4. What percentage of body weight reduction would be an appropriate goal for an obese hypertension patient?

   a. 5%

   b. 10%

   c. 15%

   d. 20%

5. Which of the following is most popular for home monitoring of blood pressure?

   a. Mercury sphygmomanometer

   b. Aneroid sphygmomanometer

   c. Auscultatory electronic devices

   d. Oscillometric electronic devices

6. Aneroid sphygmomanometers are preferred because they are more accurate than mercury sphygmomanometers.

   a. True

   b. False

7. Which of the following is true of Home Blood Pressure values?

   a. They are generally lower than physician office measurements.

   b. They are generally higher than physician office measurements.

   c. They should be about the same as those obtained in the office.

8. Patients with irregular heart rhythms are good candidates for HBP monitoring.

   a. True

   b. False

9. The finger BP monitor is recommended for Home Blood Pressure monitoring due to its ease of use.

   a. True

   b. False

10. Home blood pressure monitoring may improve adherence to therapy.

    a. True

    b. False

11. In an overweight patient, the following must be considered:

    a. A cuff that is too small may result in falsely elevated blood pressure readings.

    b. The target blood pressure in obese or overweight patients is higher than for normal weight patients.

    c. Both a and b

12. Color-coded medication schedules and picture charts are particularly useful educational approaches for which patients?

    a. Physically impaired

    b. Elderly

    c. Illiterate

    d. All patients

13. Evaluating resources on hypertension is important since some contain unproven information.

    a. True

    b. False

Chapter 8

1. Which of the following should be assessed when evaluating the clinical response to hypertension therapy?

    a. Lifestyle modification

    b. Target organ damage

    c. Patient's ability to pay for therapy

    d. Both a and b

2. According to JNC 7 guidelines, how often should followup be in patients with uncontrolled hypertension?

    a. Weekly until goal is achieved

    b. Bi-weekly for 3 months then monthly

    c. Monthly for most, more often for patients with stage 2 hypertension or with complicating comorbid conditions

    d. Bi-monthly

3. Which of the following is true?

    a. Ambulatory measurement of blood pressure has the advantage of decreasing the "white coat" effect.

    b. Clinic measurement of blood pressure is underutilized.

    c. Home measurement is not recommended.

    d. Home blood pressures are less reliable in predicting patient risk than office measurements.

4. All of the following should be included as part of periodic assessment of target organ damage except

    a. Evaluation of creatinine clearance

    b. Urinalysis for protein or albumin in the urine

    c. EKG

    d. Angiography

5. Which of the following is true?

    a. Patients with stage 1 hypertension should be started on a thiazide-type diuretic unless contraindications exist.

    b. Patients with stage 2 hypertension should begin treatment with triple antihypertensive therapy.

    c. Patients with diabetes should receive a loop diuretic since these patients usually have renal dysfunction.

6. Which hypertension patients are at higher risk for non-adherence?

    a. Patients who understand the disease and its complications

    b. Patients with co-morbid conditions

    c. Obese

    d. Patients on a complex medication regimen

7. Patients are considered to have "resistant hypertension" if they fail to achieve their blood pressure goal despite treatment with how many antihypertensive medications?

    a. 1

    b. 2

    c. 3

    d. 4

LO is a 60-year-old Hispanic male with a history of diabetes mellitus, hypertension, and hyperlipidemia. His current medications include enalapril 20 mg QD, HCTZ 25 mg QD, atorvastatin 40 mg QD, ASA 325 mg QD, glyburide 10 mg QD, and metformin 1000 mg BID. He reports that he has incorporated many of the suggestions for dietary modification that he received at the last visit. He has been able to loose 3 pounds since the last visit. He has not been able to quit smoking, which he attributes to the fact that his mother passed away shortly before the quit day he had set. The home blood pressure measurements average 150/90. He reports excellent blood glucose control and denies any episodes of hypoglycemia. Blood pressure today is 155/89, pulse 90 beats per minute. His weight is 95 kg at a height of 175 cm.

8. What other recommendations should be discussed today?

    a. Many patients need more than one attempt to quit smoking, and he should set another quit date.

    b. Weight loss measures should be continued.

c. He should not check home blood glucose anymore since readings are good, but instead focus on measuring home blood pressures.

d. Both a and b

9. What laboratory tests should be ordered today if they have not been done recently?

a. HbA1c

b. Lipid panel

c. Liver function tests

d. Fasting blood glucose

e. a, b, and c

f. b, c, and d

10. When should LO return for a followup appointment?

a. In one week

b. In two weeks

c. In one month

d. In three months

Chapter 9

1. Specialists that may be needed by hypertension patients due to target organ damage include all of the following specialties *except*

   a. Neurology

   b. Cardiology

   c. Gastroenterology

   d. Nephrology

2. Of the following roles, a pharmacist can most appropriately contribute to the care of a hypertensive patient by

   a. Ensuring appropriate dietary intake of potassium

   b. Ensuring salt exclusion in the diet

   c. Identifying opportunities for reducing costs and/or improving efficacy associated with a specific drug therapy

   d. Identifying local organizations or governmental programs that can assist low income patients

3. The pharmacist is in the ideal position to serve as the central communication link among the growing network of health care providers involved in the care of hypertension patients.

   a. True

   b. False

4. A pharmacist should call the emergency treatment services of his/her community if any of the following are detected in the treatment of a hypertension patient *except*

   a. Unstable angina pectoris

   b. Evidence of renal function deterioration

   c. Eclampsia

   d. Sudden right-sided weakness

   e. Longstanding lower extremity edema in a patient on amlodipine

5. All emergencies involving hypertension patients are most effectively treated in the hospital setting.

   a. True

   b. False

6. The Health Insurance Portability and Accountability Act (HIPAA) only affects practitioners within a hospital setting.

   a. True

   b. False

7. Patient education programs have been demonstrated to have minimal impact on patient compliance with their medication regimens.

   a. True

   b. False

Chapter 10

1. A cheaper medication is usually more cost effective than a more expensive one.

   a. True

   b. False

2. Formulary decisionmakers benefit from being able to conduct pharmacoeconomic analyses because

   a. It allows them to calculate the actual cost of therapy.

   b. It allows them to learn about new indications for therapy.

   c. It allows them to determine the most cost-effective therapy.

   d. It allows them to target new populations for therapy.

3. Outcomes research evaluated health care services in terms of all of the following consequences *except*

   a. Clinical

   b. Metabolic

   c. Humanistic

   d. Economic

4. Outcomes research can be done utilizing all of the following *except*

   a. Retrospective chart review

   b. Prospective clinical studies

   c. Computer modeling trials

   d. Patient interviews

5. Pharmacoeconomic analyses can be done to evaluate the cost effectiveness of disease state management pathways.

   a. True

   b. False

6. Pharmacoeconomic analyses can include measures such as

   a. Scores on a pain scale

   b. Cost of illness

   c. Cost minimization

   d. Both b and c

7. In decision analysis, the following steps need to occur *except*

   a. Outlining the various decisions that may occur

   b. Identifying the outcome of each decision

   c. Assigning a value to each outcome

   d. Randomizing a group of patients to each decision tree branch

8. In decision analysis, the final step should be a sensitivity analysis.

   a. True

   b. False

Index

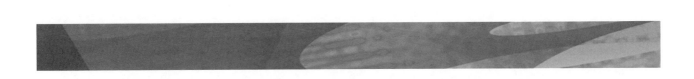

F

G

H

I

T

U

V

W

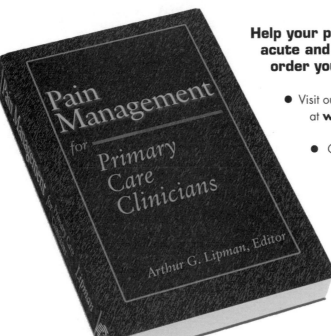
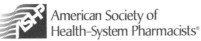

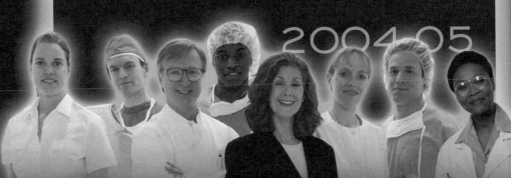